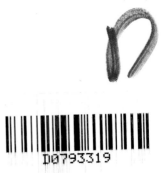

Fusion Workouts

Fitness, Yoga, Pilates, and Barre

Helen Vanderburg

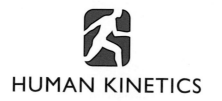

HUMAN KINETICS

Library of Congress Cataloging-in-Publication Data

Names: Vanderburg, Helen, 1959- author.
Title: Fusion workouts : fitness, yoga, pilates, and barre / Helen Vanderburg.
Description: Champaign, IL : Human Kinetics, 2017.
Identifiers: LCCN 2016013184 (print) | LCCN 2016024495 (ebook) | ISBN
  9781492521389 (print) | ISBN 9781492541752 (e-book)
Subjects: LCSH: Physical fitness. | Yoga. | Pilates method. | Isometric
  exercise.
Classification: LCC GV481 .V36 2017 (print) | LCC GV481 (ebook) | DDC
  613.7--dc23
LC record available at https://lccn.loc.gov/2016013184

ISBN: 978-1-4925-2138-9 (print)

Acquisitions Editor: Michelle Maloney; **Developmental Editor:** Laura Pulliam; **Managing Editor:** Nicole O'Dell; **Copyeditor:** Annette Pierce; **Senior Graphic Designer:** Nancy Rasmus; **Cover Designer:** Keith Blomberg; **Photograph (cover):** © Human Kinetics; **Photographs (interior):** © Human Kinetics; **Visual Production Assistant:** Joyce Brumfield; **Photo Production Manager:** Jason Allen; **Art Manager:** Kelly Hendren; **Illustrations:** © Human Kinetics; **Printer:** Versa Press

We thank Heavens Fitness in Calgary, Ontario, Canada, for assistance in providing the location for the photo shoot for this book.

Human Kinetics books are available at special discounts for bulk purchase. Special editions or book excerpts can also be created to specification. For details, contact the Special Sales Manager at Human Kinetics.

Printed in the United States of America

10 9 8 7 6 5 4 3 2 1

The paper in this book is certified under a sustainable forestry program.

Human Kinetics

Website: www.HumanKinetics.com

United States: Human Kinetics
P.O. Box 5076
Champaign, IL 61825-5076
800-747-4457
e-mail: info@hkusa.com

Canada: Human Kinetics
475 Devonshire Road Unit 100
Windsor, ON N8Y 2L5
800-465-7301 (in Canada only)
e-mail: info@hkcanada.com

Europe: Human Kinetics
107 Bradford Road
Stanningley
Leeds LS28 6AT, United Kingdom
+44 (0) 113 255 5665
e-mail: hk@hkeurope.com

Australia: Human Kinetics
57A Price Avenue
Lower Mitcham, South Australia 5062
08 8372 0999
e-mail: info@hkaustralia.com

New Zealand: Human Kinetics
P.O. Box 80
Mitcham Shopping Centre
South Australia 5062
0800 222 062
e-mail: info@hknewzealand.com

E6699

This book is dedicated to
you so you can find the joy of
movement and the positive
energy that results from being
strong inside and out. You are
a powerful being.

Contents

PART I   Foundation of Fusion Workouts

1   What Are Fusion Workouts?

3

2   Getting Started

9

3   Mindfulness and Intention

17

PART II   Fusion Exercises

4   Warming Up

27

5   Standing Strength, Balance, and Flexibility Exercises

49

6   Floor Strength, Balance, and Flexibility Exercises

81

Exercise Finder

Exercise name	Warm-up	Yoga	Pilates	Fitness	Barre	Page number
3D breathing	X					13
Abdominal brace position			X			112
Back extension			X			94
Ballet squat					X	58
Ballet squat with heel raise					X	59
Bend and stretch			X			114
Breaststroke	·		X			96
Calm lake		X				154
Cat and cow stretch	X					30
Chair pose		X				54
Child's pose	X			X		29, 153
Crescent lunge		X				64
Crisscross					X	117
Cross-legged seated forward bend		X				125
Cross-legged seated twist		X				129
Curtsy squat					X	57
Downward-facing dog	X					38
Dynamic bow		X				99
Dynamic four-point stretch				X		146
Dynamic lunge hip rock				X		136
Extended side angle		X				70
Front-lying position				X		93
Full roll-up			X			103
Fusion sun salutation flow 1	X					45
Fusion sun salutation flow 2	X					46

Exercise name	Warm-up	Yoga	Pilates	Fitness	Barre	Page number
Fusion sun salutation flow 3	X					47
Half moon		X				80
Half rollback			X			102
Happy baby		X				158
Hip extension			X			98
Knee-tuck series			X			84
Kneeling side bend					X	150
Kneeling twist				X		130
Leg lift tabletop					X	113
Low lunge				X		135
Low lunge to kneeling hamstring stretch	X					34
Lunge				X		60
Mountain pose with arms reaching	X					42
Mountain pose with side bend	X					43
Narrow push-up		X				88
Pigeon		X				137
Plank	X			X		37, 82
Plank to hip drop				X		87
Plank with hip drive				X		86
Plank with leg lift			X			83
Puppy pose				X		126
Reclining abductor stretch				X		141
Reclining adductor stretch		X				140
Reclining butterfly		X				157

Exercise name	Warm-up	Yoga	Pilates	Fitness	Barre	Page number
Reclining figure-4				X		142
Reclining hamstring stretch		X				139
Reclining knee-hug stretch				X		155
Reclining single-leg hug stretch				X		156
Reclining twist				X		133
Resting pose		X				159
Reverse table			X			105
Reverse warrior		X				68
Revolving chair		X				55
Revolving low lunge		X				131
Revolving lunge		X				62
Seated butterfly		X				138
Seated cow face pose		X				145
Seated forward bend		X				123
Seated position				X		101
Seated side bend					X	149
Seated twist				X		128
Shoulder bridge position				X		118
Shoulder bridge in external rotation					X	120
Shoulder bridge with leg lift			X			119
Side balance			X			74
Side bend			X			109
Side leg circle			X			108

Exercise name	Warm-up	Yoga	Pilates	Fitness	Barre	Page number
Side leg lift			X			107
Side plank				X		90
Side twist			X			110
Side-lying position				X		106
Single-leg balance			X			72
Single-leg squat				X		56
Single-leg stretch			X			116
Spinal rotation with thread the needle	X					32
Squat				X		50
Squat with heel raise					X	52
Standing forward bend	X					41
Supported back extension				X		144
Swimmer			X			95
Tabletop				X		91
Thread the needle				X		132
Tree pose		X				76
Two-point tabletop			X			92
Upward-facing dog		X				100
V-sit				X		104
Warrior 1		X				65
Warrior 2		X				66
Warrior 3		X				78
Wide-legged forward bend					X	124
Wide push-up				X		89

Preface

I am grateful for the opportunity to share this book with you. I have dedicated my life to active living, first through athletics and dance as a child and later in fitness, yoga, and Pilates. My passion for movement and the understanding of how physical strength harnesses the internal strength of being has been the driving force behind my 30 years of training, coaching, and inspiring fitness enthusiasts, yoga practitioners, and athletes.

The human body is meant to move. I believe that being fit is not a one-time event; it is a lifestyle. It is through movement that you maintain health, function, and vitality. Achieving fitness requires both science and mindfulness. In the fusion workouts, you will experience a combination of both to give you the best results.

Fusion workouts are a complete workout system for the mind and body. This nonimpact conditioning program will define, strengthen, restore, and nurture your body and soul whether you are a new exerciser or have been working out for years. The fusion workouts are a perfect blend of the best conditioning exercises from fitness, yoga, Pilates, and dance. This effective and efficient way to train both physically and mentally will provide you with workouts to build strength, balance, mobility, stability, flexibility, and calmness. The fusion workouts consist of body-weight training exercises and are based on the training philosophy of mastering the movement of your body with ease, grace, strength, and power without the use of equipment. It is when you master the movement of your own body that you are truly functionally fit.

The fusion workouts method is not the latest trend in fitness training but rather a system of exercises that can easily fit into your life. As your life changes, the workouts can be adapted to change with your goals and needs. When your energy is high and you're driven to challenge yourself, you can choose high-intensity fusion workouts. When you need to restore and recharge, you can practice the shorter and calming workouts. With the fusion workout method of training you do not need to give up on your workouts if your time is limited.

The five-step fusion workout structure gives you a systematic approach to training. The 15 predesigned workouts provide plenty of variety and stimulation to ensure you find the workout appropriate for you. Perhaps you are just beginning on your fitness journey or maybe you are already a regular exerciser; there are fusion workouts designed especially for you.

The book is divided into three parts. Part I outlines the fusion training principles so you're armed with the best opportunity for success. You will understand how the mind influences the outcome of your workouts and learn simple techniques for bringing more consciousness to your exercises and training for quicker and more effective results. You will learn how the core functions and how you can get the most from the exercises used in this training method. The breathing exercises, progressive relaxation techniques, and meditation described in chapter 3 are simple and easy to fit into your daily life. You can do these exercises on their own or as part of your fusion workout. You can perform the breathing exercises anywhere and at any time throughout your day whether driving your car, working in the office, or doing household chores. Progressive relaxation and meditation can be done daily at a time that works best in your schedule.

Part II contains the exercises of the *Fusion Workouts*. This is your guide for exercises in the fusion workouts. Each exercise is illustrated and described in detail to give you the opportunity to execute the exercises properly for the greatest results. The exercises are grouped into four categories: warming up; standing strength, balance, and flexibility exercises; floor strength, balance, and flexibility exercises; and calming and restorative exercises. The fusion exercise library is a comprehensive directory of more than 100 exercises and variations to select from to keep your workouts interesting, challenging, and fun. Begin with the exercises that are easiest for you and as you gain skill and strength, progress to the more challenging variations. The more variety you put into your exercise program, the better your overall results.

Part III is your collection of fusion workouts. These workout routines are based on fitness level, workout duration, workout purpose, and the type of workout you want to do. If you are a new exerciser, begin with the shorter workouts or a workout intensity that you can complete. The workouts are described so you can choose the one that is best for you based on your current fitness level and goals. I recommend that you do a minimum of three fusion workouts per week to see results. If you choose exercises at the appropriate intensity level and include variety in your fusion workouts, you can do these workouts daily.

The appendices will help you design your own workouts using the fusion workout system. Once you feel confident with the exercises in the fusion library and the five-step fusion workout system, you can begin to choose your exercises. Using a blank fusion workout template, you can build unlimited workouts. However, if you prefer to use tried-and-true workouts, sample weekly workouts based on fitness level are outlined in appendix B.

I have been teaching and using the fusion workouts for my own training for the past 10 years, and I am still finding new ways to create challenge, build strength, be more mindful, and release tension and restore, both physically and mentally. After teaching this style of workouts to instructors and participants all over the globe, I am excited to offer you this effective and efficient method of conditioning. I hope that you enjoy it as much as I do. Enjoy your fusion workouts!

Acknowledgments

Thanks to my friends and to my family: my parents, my husband, Terry Kane, and daughters, Kiah and Sage, who have supported and encouraged me to pursue my passions and share my message. To my dear friend Karen Vouri for staying up late proofreading my chapters and all who have supported me and made this project possible.

Thanks to the dedicated team of editors at Human Kinetics, Michelle Maloney and Laura Pulliam, for inviting me to write this book. This book is an expression of the inspiration I have received from the many teachers and mentors I have had in my life. I thank you for sharing with me your knowledge and inspiration to create this book and for my successful career in the fitness industry.

With much gratitude,

Helen

Foundation of Fusion Workouts

Fusion workouts are the perfect blend of exercises based on fitness, yoga, Pilates, and dance that take a mindful approach to give you optimal results. Understanding the philosophy and training principles before learning the exercises will ensure success in your exercise program.

Core conditioning is one of the hottest topics in fitness training. You will understand how to train the core and progress through your core work. You will learn breathing techniques that will enhance your core workouts by linking breath and core engagement.

Before you begin your workout, follow the simple guidelines to set yourself up for success. Learning to set intentions and being mindful of your thoughts during your fusion workouts empowers you to take control of your health and well-being. You will gain an appreciation for how the mind affects your body and physiological systems and ultimately your results.

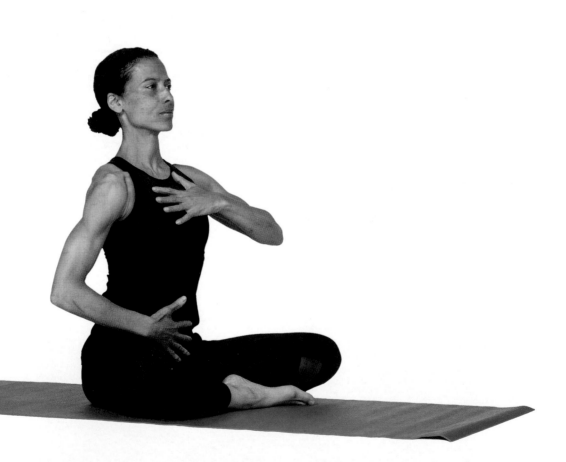

What Are Fusion Workouts?

Fusion workouts are an exciting and innovative way to get fit, build strength, change your body composition, and feel good. This unique way to train optimizes the best of a variety of exercise forms including fitness, yoga, Pilates, and barre, providing endless workout programs that are effective, challenging, and fun. The distinct blending of fusion workouts is an efficient way to gain strength, muscle definition, endurance, flexibility, and balance. And it will never get boring because the combinations of exercises are endless. Whether you want an invigorating or restoring workout, fusion workouts are versatile and will meet your daily needs.

Fusion Workouts provides a wide range of exercises and workout plans that are motivating, safe, and highly effective regardless of your experience, fitness level, or interests. Best of all, no specialized equipment is necessary—just your body!

You will learn a simple system for choosing from more than 100 exercises to create a complete workout. Mix and match the exercises to build your workout for the day or follow the preplanned workouts based on your available time, goals, interests, or fitness level.

This book will give you the knowledge to succeed by providing exercise photos, movement descriptions, and well-designed fusion workouts. Each exercise description includes simple yet effective instructions, photos showing how to perform the exercise for maximum results, and tips and modifications that make the exercise adaptable to a variety of exercisers.

Benefits of Fusion Workouts

Fusion Workouts contains a complete program for mind and body conditioning. By blending the best of yoga, Pilates, fitness, and barre, fusion workouts provide the yin and yang of mind and body training, offering both physical and mental challenges balanced with a sense calmness and restoration. This nonimpact program will define, strengthen, restore, and nurture your body and soul.

A unique feature of fusion workouts is the variety of exercise sequences that challenge the body to adapt and change, leading to incredible results and a leaner, more sculpted physique. By frequently changing the type of exercises, the sequencing, and the intensity of the work, the body is continually stimulated to make changes, producing better results over time. It is well documented that regularly changing your exercise routine keeps the body adapting and helps you avoid exercise plateaus.

Functional training is a buzzword in the fitness industry. The movement toward better function refers to the ability to perform in your everyday life with ease, strength, and endurance. One of the best ways to train functionally is by mastering the movement of your own body against gravity. This is referred to as bodyweight training. *Fusion Workouts* is a bodyweight exercise program that builds strength, balance, and flexibility for everyday life.

The fusion methodology teaches you how to master the movement of the body to get the best results. The foundation of fusion exercises is quality of movement. Exercise experts agree that quality of movement is essential to achieving the best results. Exercises done with poor technique, alignment, and posture place undue stress on the joints and eventually cause strain. You also run the risk of not achieving the desired training results. Like any activity, the better you master the movement using ideal alignment and technique, the better the outcome.

The program outlined in *Fusion Workouts* is designed to help you overcome the three biggest barriers to exercise: time, accessibility, and boredom.

Save Time

Fusion workouts are efficient. You get the best of yoga, Pilates, fitness, and barre all in one workout. You control how much time you allocate to your workout each day. With the flexibility of the workout plans, you do not need to skip a workout if you do not have an hour to dedicate to it. Simply use the fusion five-step system and create efficient workouts in as few as 20 minutes.

Access Easily

Convenience is an important factor in keeping your fitness program on track. Whether at home, in a gym, or on vacation, you can practice fusion exercises to improve muscular strength, stability, balance, flexibility, and endurance as well as to improve mindfulness and create peace of mind. With no specialized equipment or experience required, fusion exercises allow you to tailor your own workouts.

Fight Boredom

Doing anything too much and for too long will lead to boredom. A benefit of fusion workouts is that they can vary as much as you would like. The fusion system is unique in that it offers more than one way to exercise, including 15 easy-to-follow workouts based on fitness level, time, purpose, and activity. You will never get bored doing fusion workouts!

Best of all, *Fusion Workouts* gives you a wide selection of exercises at various intensities that can be done every day depending on the workout you choose. In this book, you will learn how to design your daily and weekly workout plan by using the fusion system, keeping your workouts interesting and effective.

Principles of Fusion Workouts

The three principles of the fusion workouts are alignment, movement, and breath. When you incorporate all three principles, you will achieve greater results by learning to move your body with greater awareness. Through the practice of these principles, you will gain more benefit from each exercise you perform.

Alignment

The body has an ideal alignment and posture that enables you to move with ease, strength, purpose, and grace. When the bones, joints, connective tissue, and muscles are in symmetry, the body is in balance. However, alignment is frequently out of equilibrium as the result of tension, lack of mobility, weakness, poor habits,

Integration of Fusion Practices

Fusion workouts blend a variety of movement disciplines—yoga, Pilates, fitness, and barre—to harvest the benefit that each has to offer for a well-balanced, total-body conditioning workout.

Yoga

The yoga postures have been specifically chosen to increase strength, balance, mobility, and stability. The control, focus, and mindfulness at the heart of yoga will enhance the benefit of each pose.

Pilates

The Pilates exercises focus on body awareness and core conditioning. At the foundation of Pilates is quality of movement, controlled breathing, and body alignment to build a stronger core and better posture.

Fitness

The fitness conditioning and flexibility exercises will complement the yoga postures and Pilates exercises. This will balance the overall training benefit for you to achieve a strong and toned physique.

Barre

Barre refers to the handrail ballet dancers use during their warm-up. Although none of these exercises are done holding on to a barre, you should strive for a dancer's grace, tall posture, and ease and precision of movement. Exercises should flow from one to another. These exercises will elevate the heart rate and increase the overall challenge.

Within each of these practices, your workout can be vigorous or calming by changing the repetitions, tempo, and selection of exercises. By combining each of these practices into one workout, you get the best that each has to offer. This is the beauty of fusion workouts.

lifestyle, pain, or injury. Whatever the cause may be, finding ideal alignment and proper posture during exercise will enhance your exercise results, decrease strain, and ultimately increase function. The fusion exercises aid in attaining proper posture by strengthening the muscles that tend to be weak and lengthening the muscles that have a tendency toward tightness. The best alignment for each fusion exercise is explained in the descriptions that follow in chapters 4 through 7. Remember to focus on mastering the alignment and the quality of the movement before performing the more challenging variations.

Movement

To get the most benefit from exercise, you want to perform the movements using good technique to expedite your results. When your body is properly aligned during exercises and the movement patterns are correct, you will move toward a stronger functioning body. Exercise should be challenging, but it should not hurt. Moving through a pain-free range of motion is essential for success. At first, the exercises may be difficult to perform through the full range of motion, but with practice, the movement will become easier, allowing you to take on the next challenge. The fusion exercise descriptions provide variations and progressions so you can find the intensity and exercise modification that will meet your needs.

Breath

Proper breathing will help build control and ease of movement during exercise and activities of daily life. Deliberate breathing techniques change nervous system responses and will increase strength when needed, activate the core, or release tension. Thoughtful breathing techniques will change the outcome of the exercise to invigorate you, focus the mind, or create relaxation. Using the fusion breathing techniques, you learn how breath and movement are linked and how effective breathing during movement will give you better results.

Fusion Five-Step System

All fusion workouts in this book follow the fusion five-step system. In each step you will learn a series of exercises and yoga poses to build multiple workouts with endless possibilities. Each of the five steps has a purpose with a desired outcome to advance you through a safe, effective, and rewarding workout.

All workouts begin with an intention followed by a warm-up and move into strength, balance, core, and flexibility, both standing and on the floor. The workout finishes by calming the body and mind.

Step 1: Intention

The fusion five-step system for workouts begins with an intention. Determine an intention by deciding on an action or desired result. Set a purpose and focus for your training. Thinking about what you want to accomplish in your workout each day and setting your intention before beginning the exercises will enhance your outcome. Setting an intention is a simple way to bring mindfulness to your workout. The focus of your intention will vary depending on your needs and your mental state.

Step 2: Warm-Up

The second step in the fusion five-step system is the warm-up to prepare the body for the actual workout. The fusion workout warm-up exercises take the body through a range of movements in multiple planes of motion and body positions, all at an intensity lower than in the actual workout. By the end of the warm-up, the heart rate and body temperature are elevated, the muscles and joints are mobile, and the nervous system is turned on to increase coordination and performance.

The length of the warm-up varies based on the intensity and type of exercises you will perform in the fusion workout. Generally, the more intense the workout, the more time you should take to warm the body. For a high-intensity workout, the warm-up should last 5 to 10 minutes.

The length of the warm-up and speed of the exercises during the warm-up vary based on your intention. For a higher-intensity workout, begin with slow movements through a full range of motion and, as you progress, increase the tempo. For a restorative workout, the warm-up can be short and the tempo should be slow and relaxed throughout.

Time of day will also affect how long you may need to warm up. Typically, in the morning your body will feel stiffer and will need more time to prepare for the workout. Later in the day, the body is warm, so your warm-up can be short and quick.

The most important factor in warming up is to consider how you feel. How you feel physically and mentally determines how long and how vigorously you warm up. If you feel stiff from previous workouts, spend more time warming the body. If your mind is not into the workout, give yourself permission to take it easy and gradually increase your intensity. If you need more time to feel warmed up, take as much time as you need. There is no harm in warming up longer. Fusion warm-up exercises and techniques are discussed in detail in chapter 4.

Step 3: Standing Exercises

The third step in the fusion five-step system are the standing exercises, which develop strength, balance, stability, and flexibility. Standing exercises are performed from a standing position on two feet (e.g., squat) or balanced on one foot (e.g., single-leg balance). As the standing exercises typically require more energy than other exercises and are vigorous, performing them earlier in the fusion workouts enables you to execute them well before you become fatigued. The standing exercises are described in detail in chapter 5 and are organized in a manner that you can progress and flow from a base exercise (e.g., fitness lunge) to variations of the exercises (e.g., yoga crescent lunge).

Depending on the number of repetitions, the exercise combinations you choose, or the duration of an exercise, you can lessen or increase the demand on the cardiovascular system and the intensity of the workout. Each exercise in this section has a suggested recommended number of repetitions or length of time to perform the exercise. Determine what is right for you and progress as you gain strength, skill, and fitness.

Step 4: Floor Exercises

The fourth step in the fusion five-step system are the exercises performed on the floor in a kneeling, planking, seated, front-lying, or back-lying body position. These exercises offer a higher degree of training for the core and upper body and incorporate flexibility. The floor exercises are presented in chapter 6 and are grouped by body position, making it easy for you to shift from one exercise to the next or to link exercises together for greater challenge.

Depending on the number of repetitions, the exercise combinations you choose, or the duration of an exercise, you can lessen or increase the demand on the cardiovascular system and the intensity of the workout. Each exercise in this section lists a suggested recommended number of repetitions or length of time to perform the exercise. Determine what is right for you and progress as you gain strength, skill, and fitness.

Step 5: Restoration

The final step in the fusion five-step system are the exercises to restore, rejuvenate, and revitalize the mind and body after your workout. These exercises are presented in chapter 7 and are slow, controlled, and calming in nature and focus on stretching, releasing, and resting. This step is as important as, if not more important than, warming the body before working out. For a complete workout, do not skip this step as the body needs time to recover from the workout.

Each of the steps in the fusion five-step system is essential for the best results. When planning your workouts, include exercises from all five steps to ensure a complete, effective, and safe workout.

Understanding the components of the fusion workout system will improve your workout experience and results. As you move further into this book, remind yourself of the three key principles of fusion workouts—alignment, movement, and breath. Practice these principles in your daily workouts. The fusion workout five-step system provides an easy-to-follow structure for your workout. Always begin with an intention, then a warm-up; perform the standing exercises followed by the floor exercises, and finish with a restorative series of exercises to complete your workout.

Getting Started

Getting started or staying with a regular exercise program is challenging. With so many distractions and commitments it can be difficult to get and stay fit even with the best intentions. In this chapter you will learn how to get the most from your workout sessions, how to prepare for success and be time efficient. Simply putting more time into working out is not the answer to long-term success…quality of exercise is more important than quantity. We will explore the most current information regarding core conditioning and how effective breathing techniques can stimulate the training of your core more successfully in all fusion exercises. Contemporary core training methods have moved beyond simply performing abdominal crunches to improve core strength. In fact, the abdominal crunch is not the most effective means to train your core. In the fusion workouts method, you learn how to actively work your core with a wide variety of effective core-focused exercises and how breathing exercises enhance your core training for better results.

Understanding Core Conditioning

Before getting started with your fusion workouts, it is important to understand how to achieve the most effective core conditioning and how breathing techniques can enhance the benefits of your core training. Learning how the core functions will help you achieve the greatest results in the least amount of time.

Posture and core conditioning are interrelated. Understanding the function of the core and using that knowledge to effectively work it will affect everything you do and change your appearance. How you carry yourself provides nonverbal communication to others. When you stand tall, you create an aura of confidence. The ability to stand tall and move well is linked to the function of the body's core.

Both in daily life and during exercise, a highly functioning core makes everyday activities and exercise easier. However, to understand the core, you may need to let go of old ideas on how to train it. In fact, the abdominal crunch that has long been the go-to exercise for core conditioning is in fact one of the least effective exercises.

Let's begin by understanding that the core is more than the abdominal muscles. The core is all of the muscles that support the trunk, including the shoulder girdle and the hips. The muscles of the core interlace and integrate with the muscles of the shoulders and legs. For a highly functioning core, you need to train the core three dimensionally and include exercises for the upper body, center of the body, and lower body. To simplify the complexity of core conditioning for fusion workouts, we look at the core in three groups—upper core, center core, and lower core.

Upper Core

The upper core is made up of the muscles of the chest and front of the shoulders (see figure 2.1a) and the muscles of the upper back and back of the shoulders (see figure 2.1b). The muscles of the upper back in particular have a tendency to be

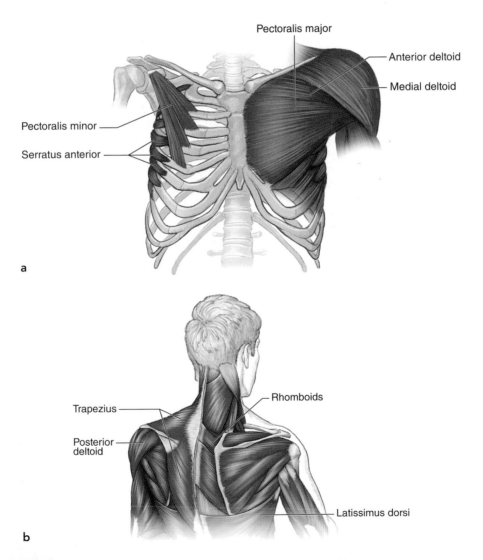

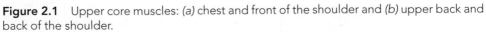

Figure 2.1 Upper core muscles: (a) chest and front of the shoulder and (b) upper back and back of the shoulder.

weak, causing a rounding of the shoulders and upper spine. Not only is this posture unattractive, but it also can cause a multitude of muscular problems in the upper back and decreases the function of the core.

When the upper back moves into a slouched position, it becomes difficult to activate the abdominal muscles, and the back muscles become strained as they try to support the bone structure—the spine and shoulder girdle—in this posture. To feel the difference in posture, try this: In a seated position, slouch the upper back and notice what automatically happens to the abdominals. The abdominal wall pooches outward and the muscles become inactive. Now sit tall with the upper body lifted and notice the change. The abdominals lengthen and move inward, and it becomes easier to contract or pull in on the abdominal wall.

The fusion exercises strengthen the muscles of the upper core and increase overall core conditioning. Pay particular attention to the alignment techniques given in the exercise descriptions found later in the book.

To find proper posture of the upper body, stand tall and bring your awareness to the upper back. Roll your shoulders back and turn the palm of your hands forward. Keeping the shoulders rolled back, move your shoulder blades toward the center of your back at the same time pull them down gently. You should feel the muscles of the upper back work to maintain this strong upper-core posture. See figure 2.2 *a* and *b* for an example of poor posture and figure 2.3 *a* and *b* for an example of good posture of the upper core.

Center Core

The muscles of the core are layered. The deepest core muscles are made up of the diaphragm, transversus abdominis, obliques, spinal muscles, and muscles of the pelvic floor (see figure 2.4a-d). This group of muscles stabilizes the core of the body and plays an important role in supporting the structures of the spine. When it comes to decreasing low-back strain, it is important to train these deep muscles.

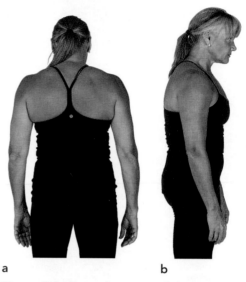

a   b

Figure 2.2 Poor alignment of the upper core: *(a)* back view and *(b)* side view.

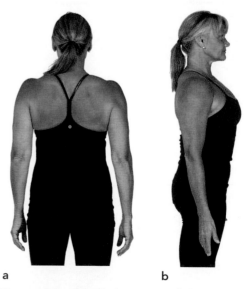

a   b

Figure 2.3 Good alignment of the upper core: *(a)* back view and *(b)* side view.

11

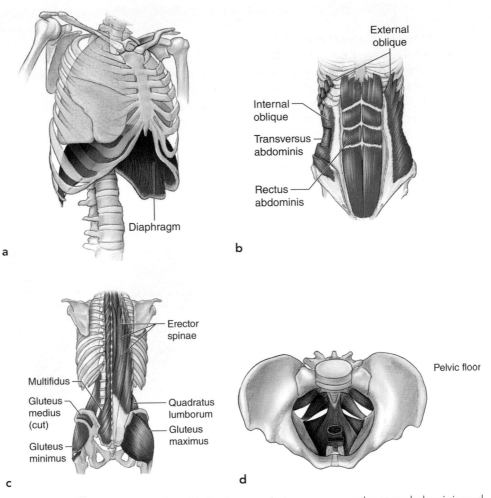

Figure 2.4   Center core muscles: *(a)* diaphragm, *(b)* transversus and rectus abdominis and obliques, *(c)* spinal muscles, and *(d)* pelvic floor muscles.

The center core can be thought of as your power center. When the center core is strong, you can generate power or muscular force in all movements from the core. Think of a golf swing. The power to make a long drive comes from the core rather than the arms. However, poor posture, inactivity, and reliance on modern conveniences can cause the center core muscles to become weak. And sitting for extended periods can cause the center core muscles to disengage just as it did when you slouched to experience the effect of poor posture in the exercise earlier for the upper core. Without intentional training of the center core, these muscles become weak and dysfunctional.

The diaphragm is considered a breathing muscle; however, because of its anatomical location and relationship to the abdominal muscles, it is also an important deep core muscle. The diaphragm is involved in core stability, and through effective 3D breathing techniques, will stimulate core muscle contraction and ultimately strengthen the core. To learn how to use the diaphragm to activate the deep core muscles, try this breathing exercise. In a comfortable, seated position, place one hand on your upper chest and the other on your abdominals (see figure 2.5).

Next, take a deep breath in through the nose and feel the chest lift upward and the abdominals move outward (see figure 2.6a). Intentionally exhale through the nose in a long, slow, controlled manner (see figure 2.6b). Feel the sensation of the exhalation begin with the lifting of the muscles of the pelvic floor, then the abdominals pulling inward and upward toward the diaphragm. Notice how this creates tension as you exhale. Repeat this breathing pattern, become familiar with the linking of your inhalation with a releasing of core tension and your exhalation with increasing abdominal tension. Try to avoid tension in any other part of your body. Observe whether your neck or facial muscles tense. If they do, you are trying too hard. The breath should feel strong, but without force.

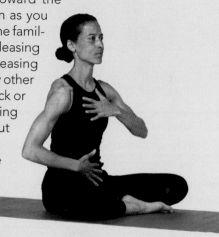

As you move into the fusion exercise series, use this core breathing technique to help turn on the deep core muscles to stabilize the spine, pelvis, and ribs. Each fusion exercise has a suggested breath pattern and can be performed in a seated or standing position.

Figure 2.5 Seated 3D breathing start position.

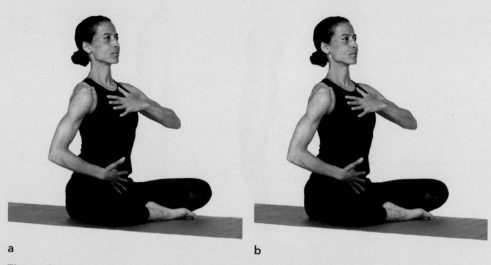

a b

Figure 2.6 Seated 3D breathing: (a) inhalation and (b) exhalation.

Lower Core

The lower core is made up of the muscles of the hips and pelvis (see figure 2.7a and b). Finding a neutral pelvic alignment will decrease pressure on the low back and hips. See figure 2.8 a through c for examples of a forward-rotated pelvis, a backward-rotated pelvis, and a pelvis in neutral alignment.

Along with the deep core muscles such as those of the pelvic floor, it is important to train the larger muscles of the hips. If you understand how to use the deep core muscles, including the transverse abdominal muscles, pelvic floor muscles, and

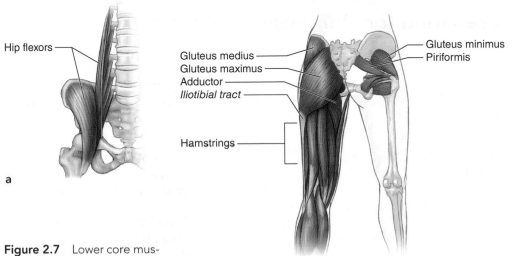

Hip flexors

Gluteus medius
Gluteus maximus
Adductor
Iliotibial tract

Hamstrings

Gluteus minimus
Piriformis

Figure 2.7 Lower core muscles: *(a)* front and *(b)* back.

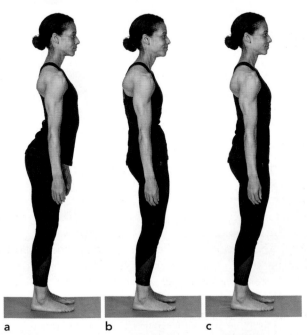

Figure 2.8 Lower core alignment: *(a)* forward rotation, *(b)* backward rotation, and *(c)* ideal neutral.

deep obliques, and then train the larger more superficial muscles, the resultant combination is a strong integrated core unit. The muscle group in the lower core that tends to be weakest in most people is the gluteals. Without adequate strength in these muscles, the pelvis can become misaligned, causing strain to the low back.

The other focus in a strong functioning core is to release the tension in the front of the hip at the hip crease. This is the hip flexor muscle group, which is often tight and pulls on the low back, increasing discomfort and decreasing core conditioning. The fusion workout exercises decrease tension through the hips and increase strength of the lower core.

Preparing for Your Fusion Workout

Preparation is an important step for long-term success. Before beginning your fusion workouts exercise program, take time to prepare yourself physically and mentally. The time spent in preparation is important for the safest, most efficient, and most effective fusion workouts. The following information provides guidelines to assist you in preparing for fusion workouts.

Consult a Health Care Provider

Before you begin, consult with your health care provider to ensure you are ready for exercise. If you have had an illness or injury or are pregnant, some of the exercises in this book may not be appropriate for you.

Ask your health care provider about health risks you should know about before starting an exercise program or that might keep you from beginning an exercise program. Once you have approval, you are ready to begin. Modifications will be provided throughout the program to allow you to accommodate injury, illness, and general discomfort.

Allow Enough Space

As you prepare for your workout, ensure you have enough space to exercise safely. Most exercises in the fusion workout program can be done in the space of a yoga mat; however, you should give yourself room to move your legs and arms to the side, front, and back.

Wear Comfortable Clothing

Nothing is more uncomfortable when you are working out than clothing that limits your movement, is too tight, or is too loose. Make sure your attire allows freedom of movement and will not limit movement. Fabric that stretches with your body and has minimal accessories such as buttons, zippers, and heavy stitching are recommended.

For women, the best choice of clothing is short or full-length exercise tights, a workout tank top, and a sports bra. For men, fitness shorts and a sleeveless or short-sleeved breathable workout top work well. Ideally, the fusion workouts are done barefoot; however, if you need foot support, wear comfortable athletic shoes.

Fuel Before and After Exercise

Be sure to eat a healthy meal or snack before you exercise. How much and what you eat is up to you and depends on several factors. Most people need one to two hours to digest a meal. A light snack that is easily digested can be eaten an hour before working out as long as it does not cause discomfort. Within 30 minutes after exercise, refuel with a combination of carbohydrate and protein such as chocolate milk. Have water available during your workout and drink frequently to keep yourself hydrated.

Gathering Equipment

The fusion workouts use minimal equipment, making them easy to do anywhere. Before beginning your fusion workout, purchase a yoga mat. Yoga mats are designed to stick to the floor, providing a safe environment for this type of training. If you find you require more cushioning, double up the mat to support the body where you feel discomfort. Other equipment that is helpful and will be used in the options and variations of the fusion exercises in chapters 4 through 7 are a yoga block, yoga belt, and a sturdy chair.

Practicing Safely

The most important consideration in any exercise program is to train safely and avoid injury. The following are a few tips to keep in mind as you get started.

- **Choose Appropriate Intensity** Fusion workouts offer a variety of workout formats and exercise selections to give you the opportunity to individualize your workout. When determining your exercise intensity, pay close attention to your breathing rate. Labored breathing indicates that you need to ease up. When performing strength-based exercises, make sure you can perform the movement using proper form and without straining. If in doubt, leave the exercise out.

- **Respect Your Body** Respect your own limitations and don't push yourself if you experience pain. If something does not feel right, make a few modifications using the suggestions in the exercise descriptions to decrease discomfort.

- **Remain Pain Free** Keep the movements within a pain-free range of motion. If you experience joint pain, stop the exercise or limit the range of motion, and gradually work toward increasing the range.

- **Challenge Yourself** Challenge yourself to improve by doing progressively more difficult exercises. When you are ready to take on the more advanced exercises or workouts, start with fewer repetitions or less time and add rest when needed.

- **Exercise Regularly** Fusion workouts can be done daily. However, if you find you are stiff and sore from a previous workout, choose easier exercises and plan for more stretching than strengthening.

Taking time to understand how to train the core and how breath and the core are linked will improve your core conditioning. Preparing for your fusion workouts and following the guidelines provided in this chapter will give you the confidence to effectively pursue your fitness goals and help you achieve the best possible exercise experience and workout success.

Mindfulness and Intention

Mindfulness and setting your intention are the foundation of the fusion workout. Lasting results and changes come from connecting the mind, body, and spirit in a way that brings meaning to your exercise program. Connecting thoughts and recognizing how thoughts affect action will increase the effectiveness of the exercises and bring fulfillment to your workout routine.

Mindfulness

Mindfulness can be described as awareness of the mind and internal sensations of the mind and body. Your mind influences your actions and your actions affect your mind. There is never a separation of the two. Your thoughts direct your actions. Your actions affect your thoughts. By learning how to set intentions and being mindful during your workouts and in life, you will achieve greater success, enjoyment, and fulfillment from your daily routines.

Connecting Thought With Positive Action

What you say to yourself matters. More and more research supports the complex relationship between the mind and body and how thoughts can change how the body functions. When the mind is stressed, the body responds by changing every physiological system to deal with the perceived stress. The obvious signals can be observed, such as an increase in heart rate and breathing frequency. However, much less obvious symptoms are changes in blood pressure, activation of the nervous system, and the release of stress hormones to combat stress. The same is true when you approach a task with self-doubt: the mind will set up the body to take on the task with apprehension and doubt. When the mind is set in a place of optimism and strength, the body and physiological systems prepare you for this outcome.

Past experiences affect how you approach a task because neural pathways in the brain have been established to respond in the learned pattern. Changing these pathways and learned patterns requires conscious effort. It is only by continuous commitment and practice that you can rewire the brain and nervous system to move you in your desired direction. Awareness of thoughts is referred to as consciousness. To develop consciousness, you must first learn to quiet the mind and body, enabling you to listen to the internal chatter of thoughts that continually flood your mind. Becoming aware of the conversations and practicing methods to redirect your thoughts will affect how you approach your workouts and your results.

By learning how to set your intentions and practicing easy yet highly effective breathing exercises, progressive relaxation, and simple meditation, you can train the mind and achieve your best outcomes. These exercises help to relax the mind and body, allowing you to replace unwanted thought patterns with new empowered thinking.

Employing Mindful Practices

In the fusion workouts, practice mindfulness to enhance your experience, satisfaction, and results. Rather than merely putting the time into your workout, practice being aware of how you feel in the exercises, the way you are performing the movement, and whether your thoughts are giving you strength and encouragement.

Three easy techniques to learn and practice to employ mindfulness are breathing exercises, progressive relaxation, and meditation. These techniques can be practiced independently from the fusion workouts or in conjunction with the exercises.

Breathing Technique

At the foundation of all mindful practices is awareness of your breath. How you breathe affects every aspect of your being. Breath is life; without it you cannot survive. Yet people take it for granted and are often unaware of how breathing affects how the body functions.

When you inhale, you bring oxygenated air into the body, supplying oxygen to the brain, organs, and muscles. The exhalation expels used air, waste, and byproducts, thereby replenishing the body through a continuous flow of breath.

Bringing Positive Thoughts to Your Fusion Workouts

Introduce positive thoughts to your practice. Powerful words or phrases will focus your thoughts in the direction you want to go. Like a mantra, repeating these words is an instrument to influence the mind. You can create your own phrases or use some of these suggestions:

I am strong.

This is my beginning.

I trust myself.

I can do this.

I am capable.

I am limitless.

If I change my thoughts, I change my outcome.

The lungs are located in the thorax and are protected by the ribs. The two lobes of the lungs are like sacks, the right side being slightly larger than the left. The diaphragm is a sheath of muscle that separates the chest from the abdomen (refer back to figure 2.4 on page 12 for an illustration showing the lungs and diaphragm). When you breathe in, the lungs fill and the dome of the diaphragm contracts and flattens as you expand the lungs into the side, back, and front of the rib cage. On the exhalation, the diaphragm relaxes, returning to its dome shape as the abdominal muscles contract inward and the lungs deflate. This action of the lungs, diaphragm, and abdominal muscles is vital for effective function of the core and all movement from the core.

In all practices, whether it be fitness, yoga, Pilates, or dance, breath is at the foundation and links to all movement. Breathing techniques can be used to do the following:

■ Increase focus and awareness internally

■ Create a sense or feeling related to the movement

■ Increase oxygen exchange to meet the demand of the activity

■ Create strength and stability in the core

■ Increase the sense of calmness and lightness

■ Relax the mind and body

A variety of breathing techniques are used in fitness, yoga, Pilates, and dance, each with a specific purpose. In fitness exercises, you are taught to exhale on the exertion and inhale on the recovery. Pilates uses a strong exhalation to assist in activating the core muscles. In yoga, the breath is linked to the natural movement of the body, the inhalation opening the body and lifting the spine and the exhalation closing the body and flexing the spine. In dance, breathing is used to find the center of the body, with the inhalation creating a strong posture and the exhalation releasing unwanted tension. At the foundation of all of these techniques is an awareness of how breath affects movement, stability, strength, and purpose.

In the fusion workouts, you will practice a specific breathing technique that draws from breath work in fitness, yoga, Pilates, and dance. The breathing method used in fusion workouts is the 3D breathing technique, which combines breathing technique from each discipline and is easily learned.

Full inhalations and exhalations revitalize both the mind and the body. When performing fusion exercises, use the 3D breathing technique to enhance the benefits of the exercises. In general, a strong exhalation will give you greater strength, and a long, slow exhalation will assist in relaxation or deepen a stretch. The inhalation fills the anterior, lateral, and posterior lungs, and the exhalation engages the core and diaphragm. This technique achieves the full potential of a breath by using more of the lungs to achieve better air exchange and activating the deep core muscles for enhanced performance and appearance.

To perform a 3D breath, follow these steps:

1. In a tall seated or standing position, place your hand on your side at the ribs. The thumbs reach back and the fingers spread along the front of the rib cage.

2. Take a long, full inhalation and feel the expansion of the rib cage under the hands (see figure 3.1a). Move your breath into the side, front, and back of the rib cage.

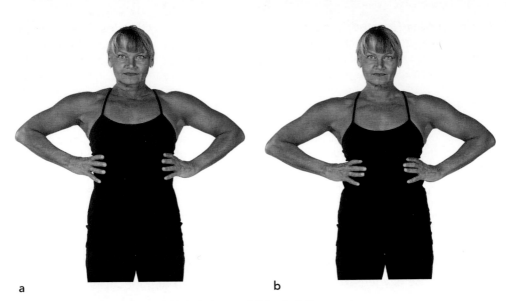

a   b

Figure 3.1   3D breathing: *(a)* inhalation and *(b)* exhalation.

3. Begin the exhalation by moving the navel inward and upward toward the diaphragm (see figure 3.1*b*). Continue to feel the contraction of the deep abdominal muscles as you complete the exhalation.
4. Repeat a deep, full inhalation. On the exhalation, see whether you can create a greater sensation of the core muscles actively working with the breath.
5. Repeat this breathing pattern without creating tension in any other parts of the body for 10 cycles of inhalation and exhalation.

Becoming Aware of the Breath

Begin by becoming aware of your normal breath and how you breathe. Spending a few moments observing your normal breathing pattern and how breathing more deeply effects how you feel will assist in learning to focus and relax. Taking the time to sit quietly and observe your breath will help you to become present in your own body and turn your attention inward. Come back to this breath awareness exercise any time throughout your day when you are feeling stressed and at the beginning or end of your fusion workout to help you to center yourself.

1. In a comfortable seated position, breathe in and out through the nose and detect where you sense the movement of breath in your body.
2. Notice the depth of your breath.
3. Observe the length of the inhalation and exhalation.
4. Take a deep inhalation and a long, slow exhalation. By changing the rhythm and depth of your breath, see how it changes the way you feel.
5. Continue breathing deeply for 2 to 3 minutes.

Progressive Relaxation

Progressive relaxation is an active method of releasing unwanted tension in the body. This technique can be done anywhere and at any time to help release stress and reestablish a sense of calmness. Before beginning or finishing your fusion workout, you can go through a series of progressive relaxation exercises. This method of relaxation is useful when you are feeling anxious and just need to release tension. Perform this simple exercise to restore a sense of well-being:

1. In a standing, seated, or lying position, begin by tensing the muscles of the entire body. Make a fist and squeeze it, tense the shoulders, facial muscles, the core, butt, and legs.
2. Inhale and hold the tension for 5 to 6 seconds.
3. Exhale and release the tension, letting go of any residual tension you are holding.
4. Repeat 5 to 10 times. On the last repetition, allow your breathing to ease back to a normal relaxed rhythm.

Simple Meditation

Meditation is a technique to create mindfulness through awareness of thoughts, responses, and action. Meditation can be done any time of the day and can be as uncomplicated as sitting quietly and observing your thoughts without action or emotional attachment. Learning to clear the mind of distractions makes room for focus, positive thoughts, and intentions to guide you with your fusion workouts. To get started, practice the simple meditation technique outlined here:

1. Sit comfortably in an upright and relaxed position. If sitting is uncomfortable, place your back against a wall or lie on your back.
2. Set a timer and begin with 5 minutes. As you practice more frequently, you can extend the time to 30 minutes.
3. Close your eyes and bring your attention to your inhalation and exhalation.
4. Move your awareness to the nostrils. As you breathe, notice the subtle sensation of cool air passing in and the warm air passing out of your nose.
5. Without manipulating your breath, simply observe. Maintain your attention to every breath with curiosity, as if each breath were your first. If your mind wanders, simply notice the distraction and patiently return to the sensation of the breath.

Intention

The first step in the fusion workout system is to set an intention for your training session. An intention is a commitment to carrying out an action or actions. Intentions require planning and forethought. In approaching each workout session with an intention, you create an opportunity to focus, build confidence and grow physically, mentally, and emotionally.

Commitment is rooted in motivation. Humans are motivated to either seek pleasure or avoid pain. In fitness training this can be thought of in terms of a need for achievement or a fear of failure. People who are motivated by a need for achievement place themselves in challenging situations that create opportunities for growth. On the other hand, people who are motivated by fear of failure may still try hard but choose less challenging tasks as a way to protect themselves. The interesting thing is that everyone experiences a level of fear, the difference lies in the ability to overcome it. This is where mindfulness and setting your intention for your workout are important. As you experience success in your workouts, you gain confidence. As you build confidence, your fears will dissipate.

Confidence is the belief in your ability to meet the demands of a given situation. Through positive experience and accomplishment, you build confidence in your abilities.

Change the way you think and feel about fear. Consider why you want to achieve your desired goals. What is your motivation and what inspires you? Create a vision in your mind of your preferred outcome or use a photo to remind you of why you are persevering. Concentrate on the benefits rather than the work. Take on an optimistic attitude and be kind to yourself. Set realistic expectations and goals to build your confidence. If you attempted an exercise or workout today but could not complete it, you are one step closer to completing it tomorrow. Focus on what you can do rather than on what you cannot. Begin from where you are today. Recognize your achievements and continue to pursue your goals.

As you approach your workouts, set an intention and challenge yourself at a level of intensity that allows success. In each of the exercise descriptions in part II, you will find helpful hints on how to focus the mind in a direction of positive action and intention.

Setting an Intention

Everyone will begin their exercise journey from a different starting place; respect that and adjust your workout based on what you need each time you do your fusion workout. Your intention for each workout can change regularly to meet your needs.

Focusing Your Intention

Setting an intention establishes the tone of your workout and directs your mind in the way you want to focus your training. This will help you focus on a specific task or outcome to help you continue to improve and achieve results. The focus of your intention can have a physical, mental, or emotional focus. Change your focus based on your needs.

- *Physical focus* is a concentration on the physical aspect of the exercises or workout, such doing a few more repetitions of an exercise or gaining upper-body strength. It can be based on a training goal such as increasing flexibility or improving balance. A physical focus can be as simple as improving your alignment during an exercise and executing the exercise to the best of your abilities.

- *Mental focus* engages the mind in observation and awareness during the exercises and workout. This can include listening to your breath and observing how your body feels when your breathing is shallow instead of deep and purposeful. It can be an internal vision of yourself performing the exercises with proper technique or an awareness of how the mind wandering affects your exercises.

▌ *Emotional focus* is paying close attention to the thoughts that float through your mind and learning to direct them and the attachment of emotions in a way that empowers you. For example, allowing yourself to experience your workout without judgment, or letting go of fear of failure during a balancing pose. Focus on a positive outcome and let go of the negative emotion attached to an exercise or workout and replace it with a positive emotion.

Creating Your Intention

To create an intention, take a moment to consider where you are today with your physical activity level, your current skill level, and your mental state. Determine the type of focus you will use for your intention by assessing your current needs. Draw from your past experiences and observations to decide on an intention. For example, perhaps you have a history of back pain and you know you need to be aware of strengthening the core without irritating your back. This experience will help you to focus your intention toward a physical goal of proper alignment and execution of the exercises. Or you may feel as though you have tried to get fit before but have failed. Turn your attention to setting an emotional focus for your intention. Use powerful and encouraging words like a mantra to overcome your past attachment to failure. At first you may not know what you need in your fusion workouts, so use the sample intentions listed here or the intentions that are suggested with each fusion workout in part III.

Sample Fusion Workout Intentions

The following sample fusion workout intentions are common focuses that can be used as your attention for your workout. You can repeat an intention numerous times until you feel you have mastered it or leave it and come back to it again at another time when you feel you need to. Listed and described are samples of physical, mental and emotional focuses.

Physical Focus: *I will focus on using the 3D breathing technique throughout my workout.*

In this case, your goal is to bring awareness to your breathing and movement throughout the workout. Observe how the inhalation lifts the torso and extends the spine. Notice how the exhalation relaxes tension in the body and moves the spine into a flexed or rounded position.

During your fusion workout, focus on how your inhalation and exhalation affects how the movement feels. For example, from a standing position, inhale and raise your arms overhead and exhale as you return your arms to your side. Repeat the exercise, but this time reverse the breath and notice how it feels unnatural.

Physical Focus: *For each exercise I will set my foundation before starting a movement.*

In this case, you want to set a good foundation so your exercises will feel stronger and more stable. For example, while standing, close your eyes and notice the weight distribution in your feet. Is your weight distributed equally on each foot? Do you feel more weight in the inside or outside edge of the foot, or more in the heel or the ball of the foot? Place equal weight on both feet and observe how shifting your weight equally between the two feet, front and back or inner and outer edge, makes you feel more stable in this position. For each exercise, set a strong foundation before moving. Continually reset your foundation to maintain better balance and stability.

Mental Focus: *Today I will focus my mind on the task at hand without distraction.*

In this case, your goal is to become aware of how your thoughts affect your ability to perform exercises. Set your intention on positive thoughts about your abilities and focus your mind on the present moment. Let go of the past and focus only on the here and now. As thoughts that distract you from the present creep into your mind, gently guide your mind back to what you are doing right now. Everyone has moments of self-doubt and negativity; if your mind drifts to an unwanted place, remind yourself that you have the power to change your thoughts. Change a negative thought by replacing it with a positive one.

An inspirational word or phrase can be used as your intention and to build strong thought patterns. For example, repeating the phrase "I am strong" or "I am balanced" in your mind as you perform the exercises will move you in this direction.

Emotional Focus: *I will respect what my body needs during my workout today and make adjustments when I feel discomfort.*

In this case, you are giving yourself permission. It's possible that inactivity, injury, or age have limited your body's freedom of movement. Set an intention to observe where you hold tightness in your body. Use your breathing, with a focus on the exhalation, to release the tension. Hold an exercise longer if the body is resisting, and gently encourage relaxation.

Setting an intention supports being mindful during your workouts. Use this technique in all your workouts and see how it helps you improve your abilities, strengthens the mind and body connection, and gives you control of your outcome. The mind is powerful. Use it to your best advantage and experience the difference it will make in your results and your sense of achievement. In the following chapters you will find suggestion for intentions and mindfulness for each of the fusion workout exercises.

Fusion Exercises

The fusion exercises are grouped in the next chapters for warm-up; standing strength, balance, and flexibility; floor strength, balance, and flexibility; and calming and restorative exercises. The exercises in each chapter will provide you the best possible outcome in your fusion workouts.

Part II contains your fusion exercises. With more than 100 exercises and variations, it is a comprehensive list of exercises to choose from to keep your workouts interesting and challenging. Each exercise has a photo and a detailed description to guide you through the exercise safely and effectively. The photo illustrates the ideal body alignment and exercise execution; however, you will progress at your own rate to master the exercise. Modifications and variations for the exercises provide you with options for intensity and ways to keep the exercise interesting and allow progress. The optimal breathing pattern is suggested for each exercise. Practice the breathing pattern while performing the exercise. Come back to this library frequently to make sure you continue to master the exercises and to add variety to your workouts.

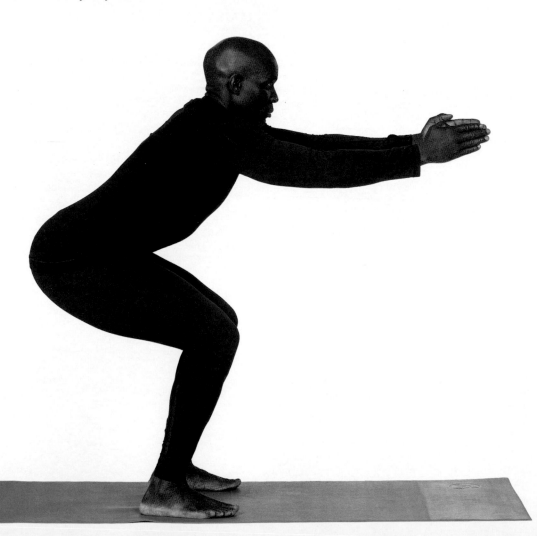

4

Warming Up

Warming the body before exercise is important for achieving comfort, mobility, and physiological readiness. By gently easing into exercise, all systems of the body have an opportunity to adapt to the work and provide the energy and neuromuscular responses to prepare the body for exercise. Movement is an internal massage to the body that decreases stiffness, increases blood flow, and warms the muscles and connective tissues so they can function with greater ease.

The warming exercises in this chapter prepare the mind and body for the workout. During the warm-up, focus your mind on your intention and let this focus lead you into the workout. Breathing helps in warming up by increasing oxygen flow throughout the body and to the brain, giving you a feeling of energy and alertness. As you learned in chapter 3, practice the fusion 3D breathing technique as you move through the exercises.

A warm-up also serves as an opportunity to gradually move into the more strenuous exercises found in the actual workout. The warm-up increases mobility, elevates the heart rate, and brings your focus to your workout. Ideally, your warm-up exercises should mimic the workout exercises, but at a lower intensity and slower speed. Depending on the fusion workout duration, type, and intensity you choose, the warm-up will vary to match the exercises performed during the workout.

Generally, the harder the workout, the longer you should take to warm up. In gentler workouts, the warm-up can be shorter because the effort required is less. Take a minimum of 3 minutes and up to 10 minutes to warm up depending on intensity and length of the workout. No matter what type of workout you do, you should always begin with a series of warm-up exercises.

The workouts outlined in chapters 8 to 11 include a selection of warm-up exercises chosen from this chapter to provide a warm-up appropriate for each fusion workout style. Exercises listed in chapter 7: Calming and Restorative Exercises can be used as warming exercises as well. In the fusion workouts you will see exercises listed that may appear in this chapter in your warm up based on the type of workout you will be performing. As you gain experience and confidence with the fusion workouts, you may begin to choose exercises from this chapter to create your own unique warm-up.

The warm-up exercises are grouped into body position to make it easy to move from one exercise to the next.

Kneeling

Warming exercises performed in a kneeling position provide a gentle way to prepare the body for exercise. In this position you are able to create mobility in the spine, shoulders, and hips as well as stimulate the core muscles in preparation for the more challenging exercises later in the workout.

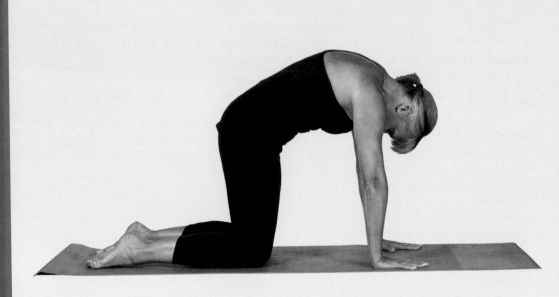

Child's Pose

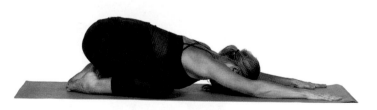

Starting Position Kneel with the tops of the feet on the floor, feet together, and the knees slightly wider than hip-width apart. Place the hands shoulder-width apart under your shoulders, fingers pointed forward.

Action Move the hips back toward the heels. Reach the arms forward and move the torso toward the floor between the thighs and knees and bring the forehead to the floor (see figure).

Alignment As you move the hips back toward the heels, keep the spine long. Avoid rounding the upper back and lifting the shoulders toward the ears.

Breath This position is ideal for focusing on breathing and creating a sense of calmness. During the inhalation, feel the ribs expand, drawing air into the lungs. On the exhalation, allow the ribs to soften and relax, allowing your next inhalation to be deeper. Hold for a minimum of five deep breaths.

Technique Tips
- Keep the spine long and shoulders soft.
- Breathing is relaxed.

Progressions and Modifications
- The kneeling position may cause discomfort or pain in the knees; minimize this by keeping the hips higher and moving the arms farther forward.
- The arms reaching forward may cause discomfort in the neck and shoulders; your option is to bring the arms beside the legs with the palms facing up.
- The forehead may not reach the floor comfortably; use a yoga block or rolled towel under the head for support.

Mindfulness Bring your awareness to your breathing and the sensation of each breath as it moves through your body. With each exhalation, allow yourself to relax more deeply into child's pose.

Cat and Cow Stretch

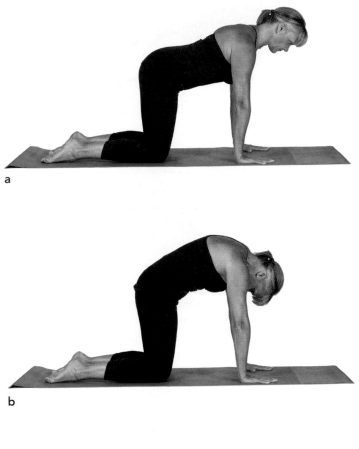

a

b

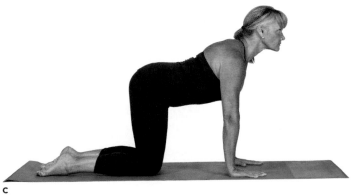

c

Starting Position   Kneel with the hands directly under the shoulders, the knees under the hips, and the spine in a neutral position. The arms are in a vertical line under the shoulders and the thighs in a straight line from the hips to knees (see figure a).

Action   Contract the muscles of the pelvic floor and lower abdominal area to rotate the pelvis under. Gradually work up the spine to the head until the spine creates a soft C-curve into cat stretch (see figure b). Reverse the action by slowly lifting the sits bones upward, rotating the pelvis, creating a slight curve in the low back and extending through the spine to the head as you go into cow stretch (see figure c). Fluidly move between the two stretches.

Alignment   Keep the arms straight throughout the exercise, allowing the movement to be experienced through the spine.

Breath   Exhale to curve the spine and gently bring the navel toward the spine. Inhale to lengthen and extend the spine. Keep the breath slow and controlled. Perform three to five repetitions of each movement.

Technique Tips

▌ Move through a pain-free range of motion.
▌ Take long, full breaths so that the movement flows with your breath.

Progressions and Modifications

▌ To decrease discomfort in the wrists, spread the fingers wide and gently press the mound of each finger (located where the finger attaches to the palm of the hand) down as you lift the palms.
▌ To decrease wrist discomfort, place the forearms on the floor.
▌ Place a folded towel or rolled mat under the knees for comfort.

Mindfulness   Observe how breath and movement are linked in this exercise.

Spinal Rotation With Thread the Needle

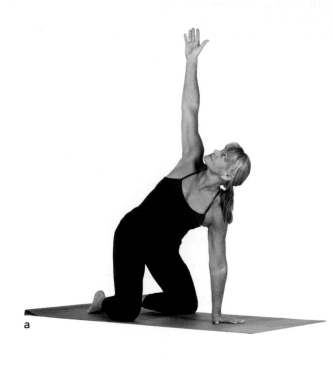

a

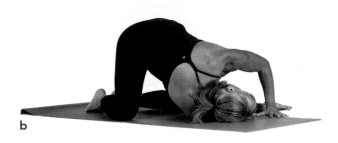

b

Starting Position   Kneel with the hands under the shoulders, the knees slightly wider than the hips, and the spine in a neutral position. The arms are in a vertical line under the shoulders, and the thighs are in a straight line with the knees slightly wider than the hips.

Action   Bring one hand in line with the center of the chest and reach the opposite arm up toward the ceiling as you rotate the spine and open the chest toward the side while looking up toward your hand (see figure a). Then bring the same arm down with the palm of the hand turned up, take the arm across the mat behind the supporting arm and toward the opposite side. Bring the outside edge of the shoulder to the floor, supporting your upper-body weight across the shoulder, and gently place the side of the head on the floor (see figure b). Repeat the exercise, flowing between each movement or choose to hold each of the movements before moving to the other side.

Alignment   Keep the hips lifted and the thighs in a vertical line to allow the rotation to move through the ribs, spine, and shoulder.

Breath   Exhale to rotate and open the chest to the side. Inhale and hold. Exhale to bring the arm through to thread the needle. Inhale and hold. An option is to hold the movement for a few breaths instead of flowing with the breath. Repeat for three to five repetitions.

Technique Tips
- Keep the thighs in a vertical position and the hips lifted as you thread the needle.
- Move from the hips to allow a fuller rotation in both directions.

Progressions and Modifications
- To decrease discomfort in the wrists, spread the fingers wide and gently press the mound of each finger (located where the finger attaches to the palm of the hand) down as you lift the palms.
- If there is pain in the knees, add cushioning by doubling the mat or placing a folded towel under the knees.

Mindfulness   Become aware of how the movement of the hips allows for freer movement in the spine and shoulders.

Low Lunge to Kneeling Hamstring Stretch

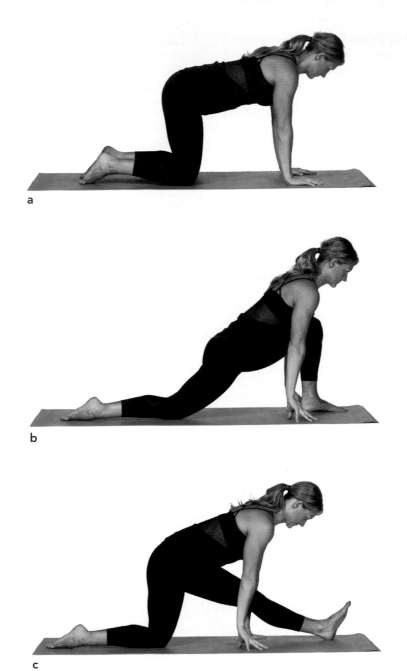

a

b

c

Starting Position From quadruped position (see figure a), step one foot forward to a bent-knee lunge with the back shin and top of the foot on the floor. Keep the forward lower leg in a vertical line with the knee directly over the heel. Place the hands on the floor on either side of the front foot (see figure b).

Action Move the hips back as you straighten the front leg and hinge the body forward, keeping the hips lifted and spine extended so that you avoid excessively rounding the back (see figure c). Allow the hips to move forward and down to deepen the sensation of the stretch. The hips stay lifted, and the supporting lower leg stays vertical.

Alignment Move forward only as far as you can while keeping the front knee over the heel. On the hamstring stretch, keep the hips lifted off the back heel.

Breath Exhale to move into the lunge. Breathe naturally as you hold the lunge. Exhale to move into the hamstring stretch. Breathe naturally as you hold. Repeat for three to five repetitions on each side.

Technique Tips

- Move from the hips between the two stretches rather than moving from the back.
- Keep the spine lengthened.

Progressions and Modifications

- In the lunge, bring the hands to the front thigh or reach overhead to increase the stretch.
- In the hamstring stretch, keep the front knee bent if there is excessive tension in the back of the leg.
- Place a folded towel or rolled mat under the knees for comfort.

Mindfulness Bring your attention to the relationship between the muscles of the legs and the hips. Observe where you feel restriction in the movement. Use the exhalation to let go of tension.

Planking

The plank body position is a foundation for many of the fusion work-out exercises. Practicing good alignment and breathing in a plank during the warm-up will prepare the body for the exercises in this body position in the workout.

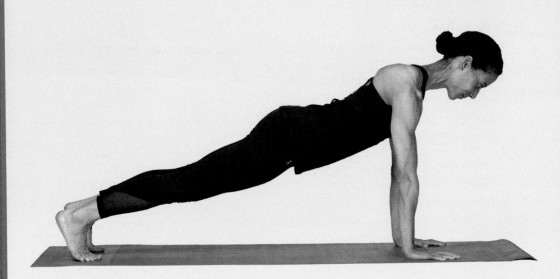

Plank Position

Starting Position   Kneel with the hands under the shoulders, stabilize the shoulders and contract the core muscles to extend one leg back, curling the toes under to balance on the ball of the foot with the heel aligned directly over the toes. Step the opposite leg back, keeping the core strong and the torso in a neutral alignment. The spine is in a neutral alignment with a slight lumbar curve and the hips in line with the spine. The head aligns with the spine. The arms are vertical under the shoulders, and the shoulder blades are drawn back and in with the chest open. Spread the hands into the floor, pointing the middle finger directly forward and the thumb reaching toward the center.

Action   Press into the hands to draw energy up the arms to the shoulder girdle. Widen the chest and bring the shoulder blades toward the midline of the back. Keep the upper body working and gently pull the deep abdominal muscles up toward the spine. Firm the muscles of the legs and lift the pelvic floor and lower-abdominal muscles upward to engage the deep core muscles (see figure).

Alignment   The spine maintains a neutral alignment, with the head in line with the spine, creating a straight line through the body.

Breath   To activate the muscles of the core, use the 3D breathing technique. Exhale to lift the abdominal muscles in and upward while creating internal tension within the abdominals. Inhale to stay strong in the exercise. Hold for 10 to 30 seconds.

Technique Tips

- Slightly tuck the chin to draw the head back in line with the spine.
- Keep the arms in a vertical line and avoid rounding the upper back.
- Maintain the alignment of the spine, hips, and head.
- Avoid lifting the hips or dropping the hips, creating an excessive curve in the low back.
- Spread the fingers wide to disperse the weight through the hand.
- Engage the muscles of the upper back and core to decrease the pressure on the wrists.
- Keep the muscles of the legs firm to support the weight of the pelvis.
- Lift the abdominal muscle toward the spine without changing the position of the spine.

Progressions and Modifications

- To decrease the intensity, bend the knees to bring them to the floor.
- To decrease wrist discomfort, place the forearms on the floor.

Mindfulness   Practice your fusion 3D breath technique to give you strength in this exercise.

Downward-Facing Dog

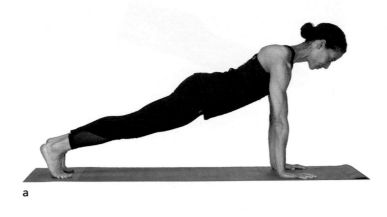

a

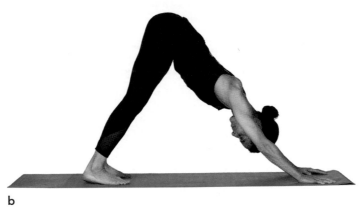

b

Starting Position   Assume a plank position, as described previously, with the hands under the shoulders, the legs straight, and the feet hip-width apart (see figure *a*). The body forms a straight line.

Action   From plank, move into a position that looks like an inverted V by lifting your hips toward the ceiling while moving the chest toward the legs (see figure *b*). At the top of the V, the arms are straight and the shoulder blades are drawn back and in to open the chest, and the heels are lowered toward the floor as far as they will go. The eyes look toward your thighs so that your head and neck stay in neutral alignment. Continue to press the thighbones back and lift the tailbone up, keeping the spine long as you open your chest.

Alignment   Avoid rounding the upper back and shifting the body weight onto the wrists. Keep the body weight moving into the legs.

Breath   Inhale to lift the hips into the pike position. Exhale to lower the heels toward the floor. Breathe naturally as you hold the position. Hold for three to five deep breaths.

Technique Tips

- To decrease the amount of weight on the wrists, lift the hips and move the legs back.
- Keep the legs active at all times by contracting the muscles to give you the sensation of the muscles wrapping around the bones.
- It is more important to keep the arms fully extended and the chest open than it is to have the heels touch the floor.

Progressions and Modifications

- To decrease discomfort in the wrist, spread the fingers wide and gently press the mound of each finger (where the finger attaches to the palm) down as you lift the palm up.
- To decrease wrist discomfort, place the forearms on the floor. Bend the knees if the backs of the legs are tight.

Mindfulness   This exercise requires both strength and flexibility. Notice the sensation of stretching and strengthening in this exercise.

Standing

The standing exercises during the warming phase of the fusion workouts provide you an opportunity to become grounded, becoming aware of the position of the feet and activation of the leg muscles. The standing position in the warm-up is the foundation for all standing exercises in the fusion workouts.

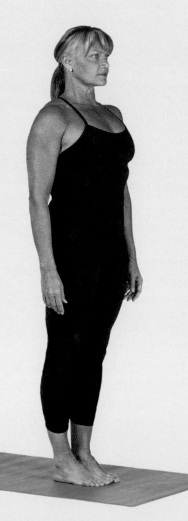

Standing Forward Bend

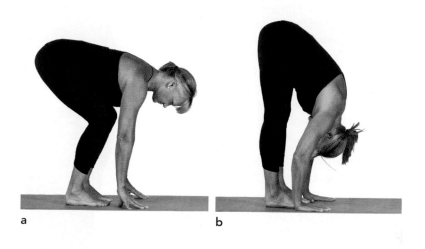

a   b

Starting Position   Support your upper-body weight with your hands on the floor or on your thighs, depending on your hamstring flexibility. Place the feet approximately shoulder-width apart (see figure a) and the feet in a parallel position with the toes pointing forward.

Action   Gently straighten the legs, lifting the hips upward and moving the crown of the head toward the floor with the chin gently tucked. Press equally into all four corners of the feet to lift the hips upward and move the torso downward. (see figure b).

Alignment   Keeping the legs active, lift the chest to lengthen the spine to create more length in the stretch.

Breath   Inhale to lift the hips upward. Exhale to fold the upper body toward the legs. Breathe naturally as you hold. Inhale to lift the chest and lengthen the spine from the hips. Exhale once again to bend into the stretch. Hold for 10 to 30 seconds.

Technique Tips

▌ Keep the upper body supported with the hands on the floor or the thighs.
▌ Think of lifting the tailbone toward the ceiling.

Progressions and Modifications

▌ Bend the knees if the backs of the legs are tight.
▌ If bending forward makes you dizzy, place the hands on the back of a chair to keep the head above the heart.

Mindfulness   Avoid holding your breath. Focus on a long exhalation to assist you into this stretch.

Mountain Pose With Arms Reaching

Starting Position   Start in a tall standing position, with feet together or slightly apart and arms by your side. The shoulders relax down and away from the ears and slightly back to open the front of the chest. The head should rest directly over the spine, with the tip of the nose pointed forward and the gaze straight ahead. The chin is tucked slightly.

Action   Raise the arms out to the side and then overhead (see figure). Lower them back to the sides.

Alignment   Keep the shoulders relaxed away from the ears as you bring the arms overhead.

Breath   Inhale to lift the arms overhead. Exhale to lower the arms. Repeat three to five times.

Technique Tips

- Keep the shoulders relaxed and down as the arms lift overhead.
- The spine and pelvis are in a neutral alignment.

Progressions and Modifications

- Bend the elbows and keep the arms slightly in front of the head if the shoulders are tight.
- Hold the arms down by your side or in a prayer position in front of the chest.

Mindfulness   Mountain pose is the foundation for all standing exercises. Focus on the feet and press them into the floor to create a sensation of lifting through the spine. Focus your attention on creating a tall posture and lengthening from the feet to the top of the head.

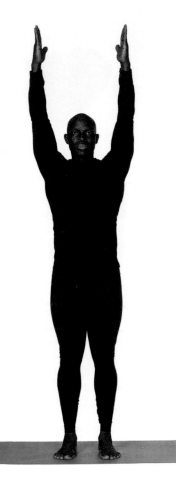

Mountain Pose With Side Bend

Starting Position Start in a tall standing position. Feet are together or slightly apart and arms by your side. The shoulders are relaxed and down and away from the ears and slightly back to open the front of the chest. The head should rest directly over the spine, with the tip of the nose pointed forward, the gaze straight ahead, and the chin slightly tucked.

Action Move the arms out to the side, bringing them overhead with the palms of the hands turned into the center, and bend to one side (see figure). Come back to the center and bend to the opposite side.

Alignment Keep the shoulders relaxed and away from the ears as you bring the arms overhead.

Breath Inhale to lift the arms overhead. Exhale to bend to the side and inhale to come back to the center. Exhale to go to the other side. Repeat three to five times on each side.

Technique Tips

- Keep the shoulders relaxed and down as the arms lift overhead.
- When bending to the side, keep the upper body straight and keep the movement lateral. Don't bend forward or round the back.

Progressions and Modifications

- Bend the elbows and keep the arms slightly in front of the head if the shoulders are tight.
- Bring the hands together overhead for a greater stretch.

Mindfulness Focus on the feet pressing equally into the floor as you bend to the side to create a lengthening of the side of the body.

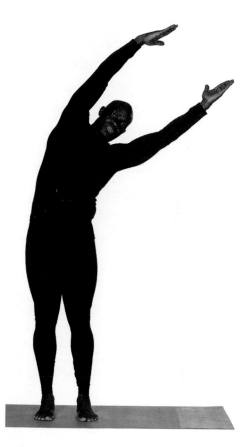

Sun Salutation

The fusion sun salutation is based on the traditional yoga sun salutation, with additional movements and modifications to allow you to choose the version that's best for you. The sun salutation links movements and breath together in a flow to create heat in the body. Each fusion sun salutation flow is progressively more challenging. Follow the guidelines for the number of repetitions of the fusion sun salutations to complete in the workouts described in Part III, Fusion Workout System.

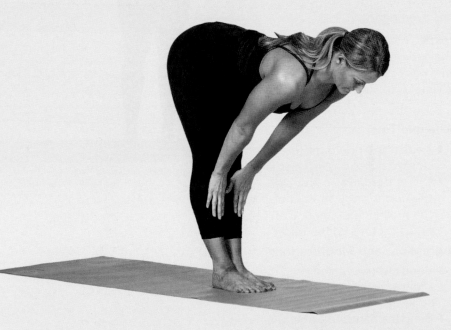

Fusion Sun Salutation Flow 1

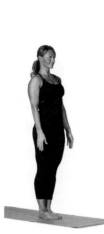

Mountain pose.

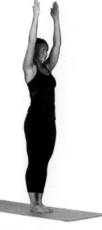

Inhale, arms overhead.

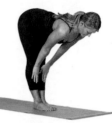

Exhale, hinge forward from the hips, bringing the hands to shins, feet, or floor. Inhale, extend the spine in a supported forward bend.

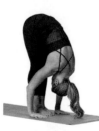

Exhale, fold into the legs.

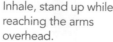

Inhale, stand up while reaching the arms overhead.

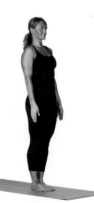

Exhale, lower the arms to the side.

Fusion Sun Salutation Flow 2

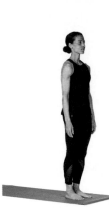

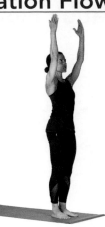

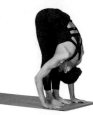

Mountain pose.

Inhale, arms overhead.

Exhale, hinge forward from the hips into a forward bend with the hands coming to the shins, feet or floor.

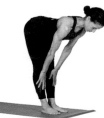

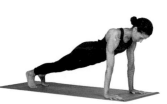

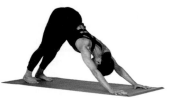

Inhale, lengthen the spine from the hips to head.

Exhale, bend the knees and bring the hands to the floor and walk feet back to a plank position. Inhale and hold.

Exhale, lift the hips to downward-facing dog (or child's pose for modification). Hold for five deep breaths.

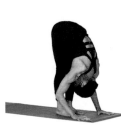

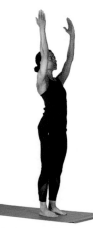

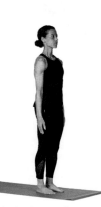

Inhale, walk the feet to the hands. Exhale, fold forward, bringing the chest into the legs.

Inhale, stand up while reaching the arms overhead.

Exhale, lower the arms to the side.

Fusion Sun Salutation Flow 3

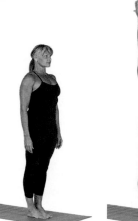

Mountain pose.

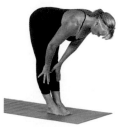

Inhale, reach the arms overhead.

Exhale, hinge from the hips to a forward bend with the hands coming to the shins, feet or floor. Inhale, lengthen the spine.

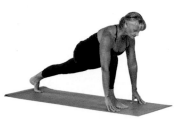

Exhale, bend the knees and bring the hands to the floor. Step one foot back and lower into a low lunge. Inhale, hold.

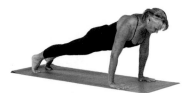

Exhale, step back to a plank. Inhale, hold.

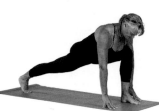

Inhale, step the other foot forward to a low lunge and hold.

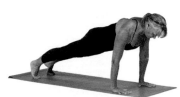

Exhale, step back to a plank. Inhale, hold.

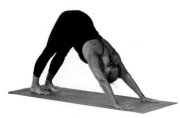

Exhale, lift the hips up to downward-facing dog (or child's pose for modification). Take five deep breaths.

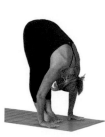

Inhale, walk or jump your feet to your hands. Exhale, fold into the legs.

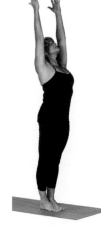

Inhale, stand up while reaching the arms overhead.

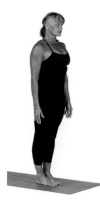

Exhale, lower the arms to the side.

5

Standing Strength, Balance, and Flexibility Exercises

The exercises in this chapter build strength, balance, and flexibility in the lower body while integrating core training. The standing exercises define the muscles of the legs, buttocks, back, and abdominals through a focus on proper alignment and posture. Because these exercises use the largest muscles in the body, the intensity of the exercises and the caloric expenditure are high. If changing your body composition is your goal, add more of these exercises to your workouts.

The standing exercises are grouped in similar movement patterns that build from a foundational movement. A foundational movement uses a body position or exercise that is common to other exercises. For example, a squat is a foundational fitness exercise that is similar in position to a yoga chair pose or a squat with heel raise, which is a barre exercise. Once you learn the position and technique required in the foundational exercise, you will use similar technique in all the other exercises that use that movement pattern. Grouping the exercises in this way makes it easy to move from one exercise to the next with minimal adjustments in body position. Not only is this more efficient, but it also assists in mastering the exercise technique. From the foundational exercises, you can choose a variety of exercise options. Using the fusion method, you will be able to easily mix and match the exercises within each group to flow from one exercise to another to change the intensity and to bring novelty to your workouts.

Squat

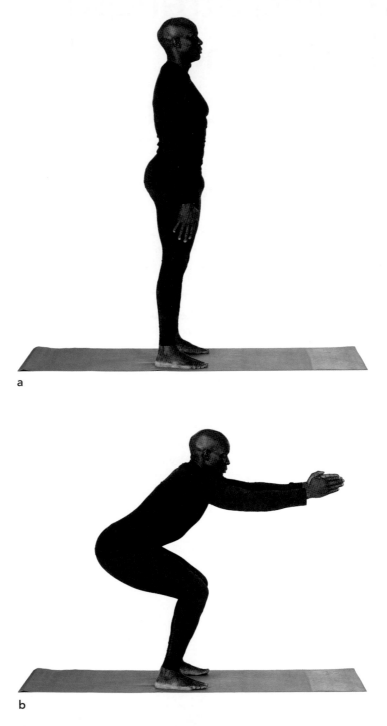

a

b

Starting Position   Start in a tall standing position. The feet are approximately shoulder-width apart and the toes point forward (see figure *a*). The knees align directly over the midline of the feet and extend no farther forward than the ball of the foot. The spine is in a neutral alignment and the head is in line with the spine. The eyes focus straight ahead, and the chin is tucked slightly. The shoulders are relaxed and down and away from the ears and the arms are by your side. The chest is lifted and opened by bringing the shoulder blades toward the middle of the back.

Action   Keeping the spine in a neutral and lengthened position, bend at the knees, hips, and ankles to lower the torso until the thighs are parallel or slightly higher than parallel to the floor as you descend into a squat (see figure *b*). Lift the pelvic floor and lower-abdominal muscles to engage the core. The torso will naturally hinge forward from the hips as you lower into the squat. Press down into the feet to push up to standing. The arms reach forward as you squat, and they lower to the side as you stand up.

Alignment   Keep the spine lengthened and torso in a tall posture as you move through the squat. The knees stay aligned over the center of the feet. Avoid letting the knees fall inward or outward as you squat.

Breath   Inhale to lower into the squat. Exhale to press up to standing, maintaining neutral alignment of the pelvis, spine, and shoulder girdle. Repeat 8 to15 times.

Technique Tips

- Keep equal weight on the balls and heels of both feet.
- Maintain the alignment of the knees with the feet to keep the knees from falling inward or outward as you lower into the squat.
- Hinge or sit back with the hips as you lower into the squat.
- Keep the chest lifted and the spine long throughout the movement.
- Relax the shoulders down and away from the ears.
- Maintain the head's neutral alignment with the spine.

Progressions and Modifications

- Hold the bottom of the squat longer for more intensity.
- Increase the range of motion by moving deeper into the squat.
- Stand higher in the squat to decrease the intensity.

Mindfulness   Control your breathing to give you strength in this challenging exercise. Take a strong breath in as you lower into the squat, and exhale to push up to standing.

Squat With Heel Raise

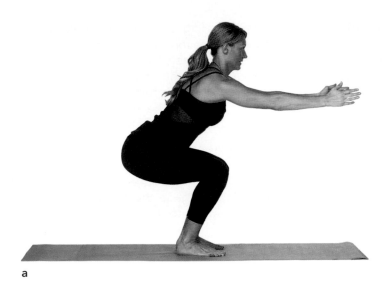

a

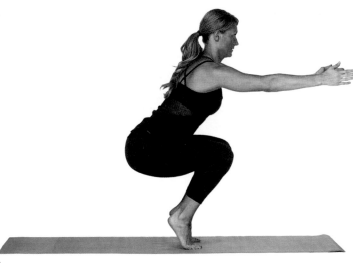

b

Starting Position   Start in a tall standing position, with the feet approximately shoulder-width apart and the toes pointing forward. Align the knees directly over the midline of the feet and extend no farther forward than the ball of the foot. The spine is in a neutral alignment and the head is in line with the spine. Focus the eyes straight ahead, and the tuck the chin slightly. The shoulders are relaxed and down and away from the ears and the arms are by your side. Lift and open the chest by bringing the shoulder blades toward the middle of the back.

Action   Lower into the squat (see figure a); at the bottom, lift both heels, balancing on the balls of the feet (see figure b). Lower the heels and stand up. Reach the arms in front of the shoulders to help you balance as you lift and lower the heels.

Alignment   Keep the knees in line with the toes as you lower into the squat and as you lift and lower the heels. The weight should stay centered across the balls of the feet. Avoid rolling the ankles in or out.

Breath   Exhale to lower into the squat, inhale to lift the heels, exhale to lower the heels, and inhale to stand up. Repeat 5 to15 times.

Progressions and Modifications
- To add intensity, stay at the bottom of the squat, and lift and lower the heels for three to five repetitions.
- To assist with balance, hold the back of a chair.

Mindfulness   Use strong breathing to help you through this challenging exercise. Focus your eyes on a single point to assist with balance.

Chair Pose

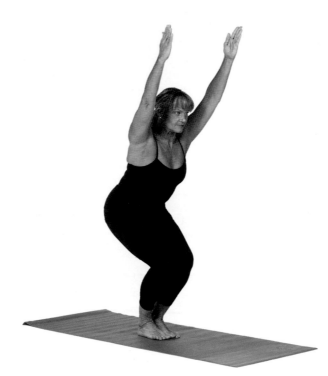

Starting Position   Stand tall with the feet together or shoulder-width apart.

Action   Lower into a squat, hold the bottom of the squat, and bring the arms overhead in line with the ears (see figure).

Alignment   Keep the spine in a neutral alignment, the chest open, and the shoulders relaxed down and away from the ears.

Breath   Exhale to lower into the squat, and inhale to lift the arms. Hold for three to five breaths before standing up.

Progressions and Modifications
- To increase the balance challenge, place the feet together.
- To decrease the balance challenge, place the feet hip-width apart.
- To add intensity, stay in chair pose for more than five breaths.
- To decrease the challenge, keep the hips higher.

Mindfulness   Bring your attention to the core muscles, particularly the abdominal muscles. Consciously lift the abdominal wall up and away from the thighs to support the low back.

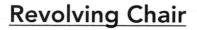

Revolving Chair

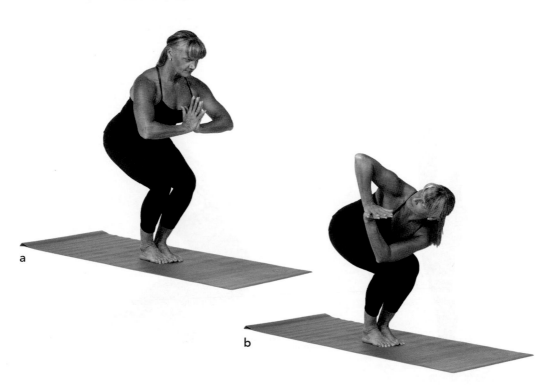

a

b

Starting Position   Stand tall with the feet together or shoulder-width apart.

Action   Lower into a squat, hold the bottom of the squat, and bring the hands together in a prayer position in front of the chest (see figure *a*). Keeping the hips square and the knees aligned, bring an elbow across to the opposite thigh as you rotate the upper body (see figure *b*).

Alignment   Keep the weight equal on both feet and the knees aligned with each other as you twist to the side.

Breath   Exhale to lower into the squat, and inhale as you lift the arms. Exhale as you rotate to one side. Hold for three to five breaths. Inhale to return to center. Exhale to stand up. Repeat on the other side.

Progressions and Modifications
- To increase the balance challenge, move the feet together.
- To decrease the balance challenge, move the feet hip-width apart.
- To add intensity, stay in revolving chair for more than five breaths.
- To decrease the challenge, position the hips higher.

Mindfulness   Soften the tension in the body and the mind by using a long slow exhalation to rotate. Keep the mind peaceful as you hold the pose.

Single-Leg Squat

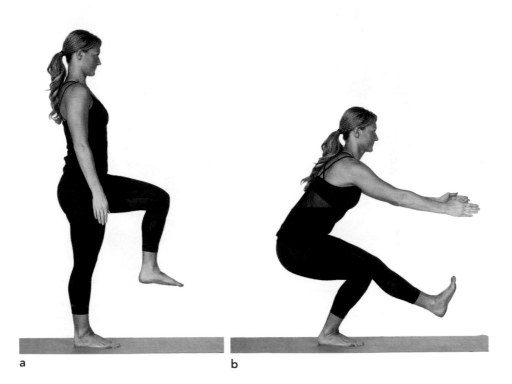

a   b

Starting Position   Stand tall and press into one foot to lift the opposite foot so you are balancing on one leg (see figure a).

Action   Keeping the foot lifted, bend the knee of the supporting leg as your hips lower into a squat (see figure b). Press up to the single-leg balance.

Alignment   Keep the knee centered over the foot and your body weight back into the hips as you lower into the squat.

Breath   Exhale to lower into the squat. Inhale to hold the bottom of the squat. Exhale to stand up. Complete five to eight repetitions per side.

Progressions and Modifications

- To add intensity, complete more repetitions or increase the depth of the squat.
- To assist with balance, place your hands on the back of a chair or the wall.

Mindfulness   Focus your attention on grounding the supporting foot into the floor to give you a stronger foundation for this balance exercise. Think of the foot growing roots into the floor.

Curtsy Squat

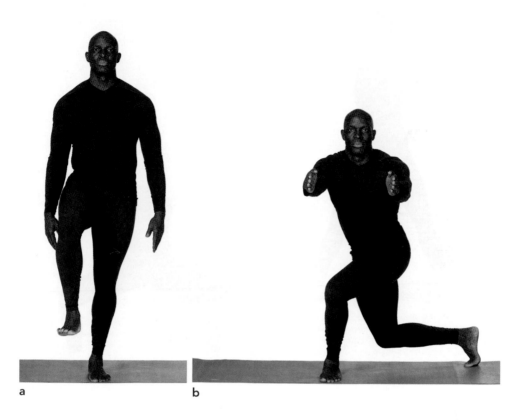

a   b

Starting Position   Press down on to one foot and lift the opposite foot so you are balancing on one leg (see figure a).

Action   Keeping the foot lifted, lower into the squat, crossing the lifted leg diagonally behind you to touch the toe on the floor (see figure b). Press up to the standing balance.

Alignment   Keep the shoulders and hips facing forward as you cross the leg behind in the curtsy. The front knee stays aligned over the center of the foot.

Breath   Exhale to lower into the squat. Inhale to hold the bottom of the squat. Exhale to stand up. Complete five to fifteen repetitions per side.

Progressions and Modifications

- To add intensity, complete more repetitions or increase the depth of the squat.
- To add more range of motion and core conditioning, add a rotation of the upper body and arms as you squat. Rotate to the same side as the back leg.
- To assist with balance, place your hands on the back of a chair or the wall.

Mindfulness   This exercise challenges both strength and balance, so keep your thoughts positive and your mind focused on feeling graceful.

Ballet Squat

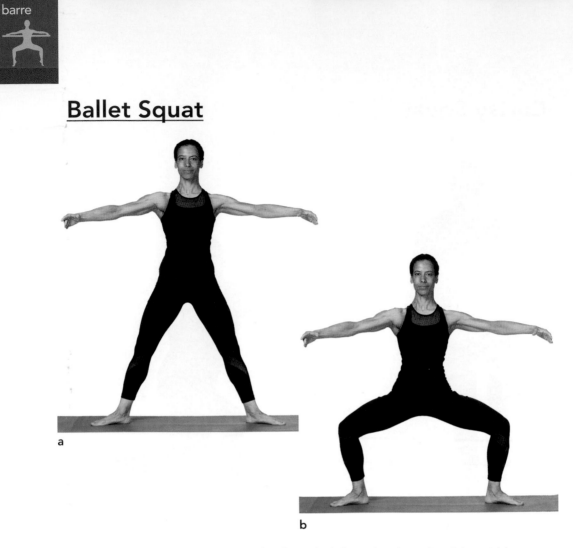

a

b

Starting Position   Stand with the feet slightly wider than shoulder-width apart, externally rotate the hips to point the toes out, and keep the knees aligned over the feet (see figure a). The pelvis is in a vertical position and the rib cage centered over the hips. Lift the pelvic floor and lower-abdominal muscles to engage the core.

Action   Lower into the ballet squat, keeping the torso and pelvis in a neutral alignment and the tailbone pointing down (see figure b). Press up and straighten the legs to full standing without hyperextending the knees.

Alignment   At the bottom of the squat, the knees should not extend beyond the toes. Keep equal pressure on the inside and the outside edges of the feet.

Breath   Inhale to set the core, and exhale to lower in the ballet squat. Inhale to hold the bottom. Exhale to stand up. Complete 8 to 15 repetitions.

Progressions and Modifications

> ▍ To add intensity, complete more repetitions.
> ▍ To assist with balance, hold on to the back of a chair.

Mindfulness   Feel the movement from the hips and as you lower and lift, keep the hips rotating outward to maintain the alignment of the knees. Imagine the big toes pressing into the floor and the thigh rolling outward.

Ballet Squat With Heel Raise

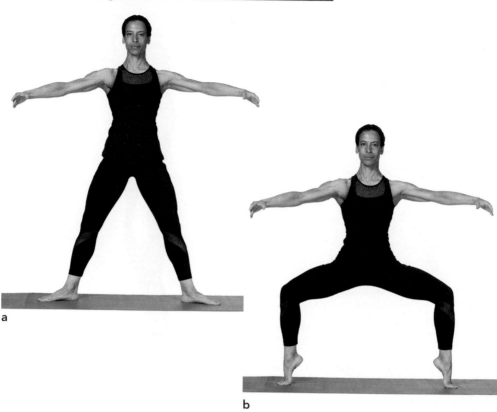

a

b

Starting Position Stand with the feet slightly wider than shoulder-width apart, externally rotate the hips to point the toes out, and keep the knees aligned over the feet (see figure *a*). The pelvis is in a vertical position, and the rib cage is centered over the hips. Lift the pelvic floor and lower-abdominal muscles to engage the core.

Action Lower into the ballet squat, keeping the torso and pelvis in a neutral alignment and the tailbone pointing down, and lift the heels (see figure *b*). Lower the heels. Press up and straighten the legs to full standing.

Alignment At the bottom of the squat, the knees should not extend beyond the toes. Maintain equal pressure on the inside and the outside edges of the feet.

Breath Inhale to set the core, and exhale to lower into the ballet squat. Inhale to lift the heel, and exhale to lower and stand up. Complete 8 to 12 repetitions.

Progressions and Modifications

- To add intensity, complete more repetitions or hold the bottom of the squat and perform repetitive heel lifts.
- To assist with balance, place your hands on the back of a chair or the wall.

Mindfulness As you lift and lower the heel, feel the control come from your core and lift the pelvic floor to control the movement of the feet.

Lunge

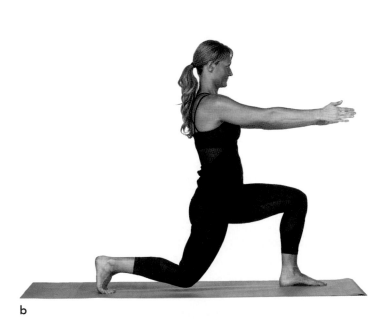

a

b

Starting Position   Stand tall with the feet hip-width apart and the knees aligned directly over the center of the feet. Maintain a neutral alignment of the spine. The shoulders are relaxed down and away from the ears and slightly back to open the front of the chest (see figure a).

Action   Step one leg behind you and bend the front knee to just above 90 degrees. The knee is directly over the ankle. At the same time, bend the back knee toward the floor while maintaining neutral spinal alignment (see figure b). Keep the pelvis and spine in a neutral position and the ribs over the hips. Engage the core muscles to maintain a neutral spine as you press the feet into the floor to push up to standing. The arms reach to the front or to the side for balance. Press up by straightening the legs.

Alignment   Keep the knees aligned directly over the center of the feet. Maintain a neutral alignment of the spine. The shoulders are relaxed down and away from the ears and slightly back to open the front of the chest.

Breath   Exhale to press up to standing, maintaining neutral alignment of the pelvis, spine, and shoulder girdle. Inhale to lower. Repeat 8 to 15 times per side.

Technique Tips

- Press equally into the ball and heel of the front foot.
- The back heel is lifted off the floor throughout the exercise, and the heel is over the ball of the foot.
- Keep the knees aligned over the feet; avoid letting the knees fall inward or outward.
- The hips should move up and down in a vertical line.
- Keep the chest lifted and the spine long throughout the movement.
- Relax the shoulders down and away from the ears.
- The head is in a neutral alignment with the spine.

Progressions and Modifications

- Change the tempo of the lunge by lowering and rising at different rhythms: two counts up and down, four counts up and down, three counts down and one count up, or one count down and three counts up.
- To add intensity, add an isometric (not moving) hold at the bottom of the lunge for two to eight counts before standing and repeat.
- Stand higher in the lunge to decrease the intensity.

Mindfulness   Observe how one side feels compared to the other. Is there more tension or less strength or balance on one side of the body than the other? If one side is weaker, spend more time practicing the exercise on that side of the body to equalize the two sides.

Revolving Lunge

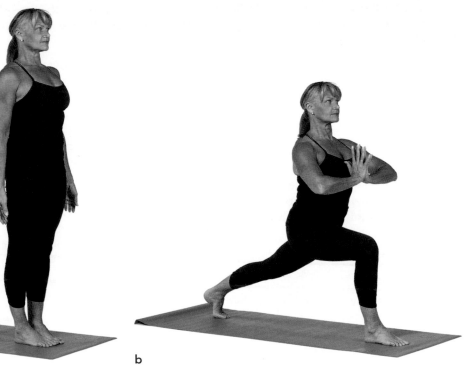

a

b

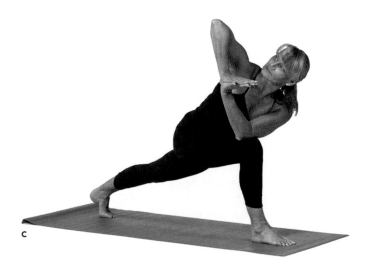

c

Starting Position   Stand tall with the feet hip-width apart and the knees aligned directly over the center of the feet. Maintain a neutral alignment of the spine. The shoulders are relaxed down and away from the ears and slightly back to open the front of the chest (see figure *a*).

Action   Step one leg behind you and bend the front knee to just above 90 degrees (see figure *b*). The knee is directly over the ankle. Keep the back leg straight and the ball of the foot on the floor and the heel lifted. Bring the hands together in a prayer position in front of the chest. Hinge the torso forward and bring the opposite elbow across the front thigh by initiating the rotation from the hips through the top of the head (see figure *c*). Place the elbow on the opposite thigh. Fingertips point forward and the gaze is toward the top elbow.

Alignment   Keep the back foot grounded and initiate the rotation from the back leg by rolling the leg in. Finish the rotation through the ribs, spine, and shoulders, giving you a sense of rotation through the entire body.

Breath   Inhale to hinge forward. Exhale to rotate into the revolving lunge. Breathe naturally and relax unwanted tension. Hold for three to five breaths per side.

Progressions and Modifications

- To increase intensity, lower the hips to form a 90-degree angle in the front knee.
- To move deeper into the twist, open the arms out by reaching one hand down and the other up.
- Stand higher in the lunge to decrease the intensity.
- If the rotation is too challenging, place your supporting hand on the thigh and the opposite hand on the hip.

Mindfulness   Bring awareness to your breathing. Your breath should flow freely and deeply as you rotate. If your breath becomes restricted, create more length in the spine and open the chest.

Crescent Lunge

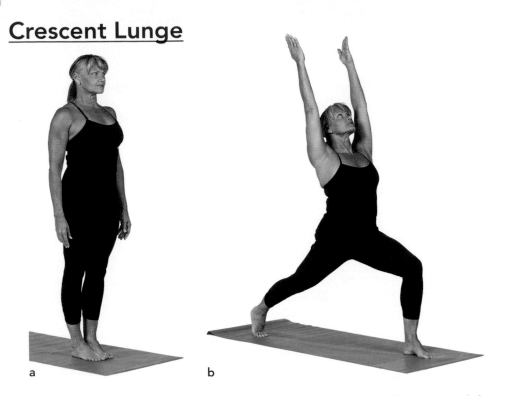

a   b

Starting Position Stand tall with the feet together or hip-width apart and the knees aligned directly over the center of the feet. Maintain a neutral alignment of the spine. The shoulders are relaxed down and away from the ears and slightly back to open the front of the chest (see figure *a*).

Action Step one leg behind you and bend the front knee to just above 90 degrees. The knee is directly over the ankle. Keep the back leg straight, the ball of the foot on the floor, and the heel lifted. Raise both arms overhead with the palms facing each other (see figure *b*). Engage the core muscles to maintain a neutral spine position.

Alignment Align the pelvis and spine in a neutral position and the ribs over the hips. Engage the core muscles to maintain a neutral spine.

Breath Inhale to reach the arms overhead. Exhale to relax unwanted tension in this exercise. Hold for three to five breaths per side.

Progressions and Modifications

- To increase intensity, lower the hips to form 90-degree angle in the front knee.
- To add an upper-body stretch, reach the arms behind the back and interlace the fingers. With the arms straight, lift the hands upward to open the front of the shoulder and chest.
- Stand higher in the lunge to decrease the intensity.
- To move into a deeper stretch, bring your hands to the floor for a low lunge.
- For better balance, reach the arms in front of the chest and look forward.

Mindfulness Focus on the position of the hips. Keep the hips level under the shoulders. As you rotate the tailbone downward, notice the increase in the stretch in the front of the hip of the back leg.

Warrior 1

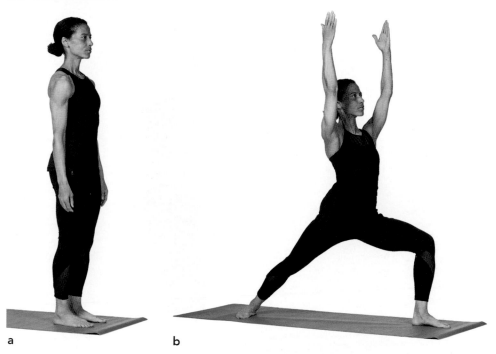

a   b

Starting Position Stand tall with the feet together or hip-width apart and the knees aligned directly over the center of the feet. Maintain a neutral alignment of the spine. The shoulders are relaxed down and away from the ears and slightly back to open the front of the chest (see figure a).

Action Step one leg behind you and bend the front knee to just above 90 degrees, lined up directly over the ankle. Keep the back leg straight. Lift onto the ball of the back foot and rotate the hips outward to turn the heel of the foot in and down. Press into the outside edge of the back foot, lift through the thigh, and rotate the hip toward the front. Lift the pelvic floor and lower-abdominal muscles to engage the core to maintain a neutral spine. Raise both arms overhead with the palms facing each other (see figure b).

Alignment With the back hip and foot rotated out, keep the hips and torso rotating toward the front. Keep the shoulders relaxed down and away from the ears and slightly back to open the front of the chest as you lift the arms.

Breath Inhale to reach the arms overhead. Exhale to relax unwanted tension as you hold for three to five breaths per side.

Progressions and Modifications

- Step the back foot out to the side to widen the stance if there is discomfort in the hips or back and to help with balance.
- Stand higher in the lunge to decrease the intensity.

Mindfulness Focus on the position of the hips. As you rotate the tailbone downward, notice the increase in the stretch in the front of the hip of the back leg.

Warrior 2

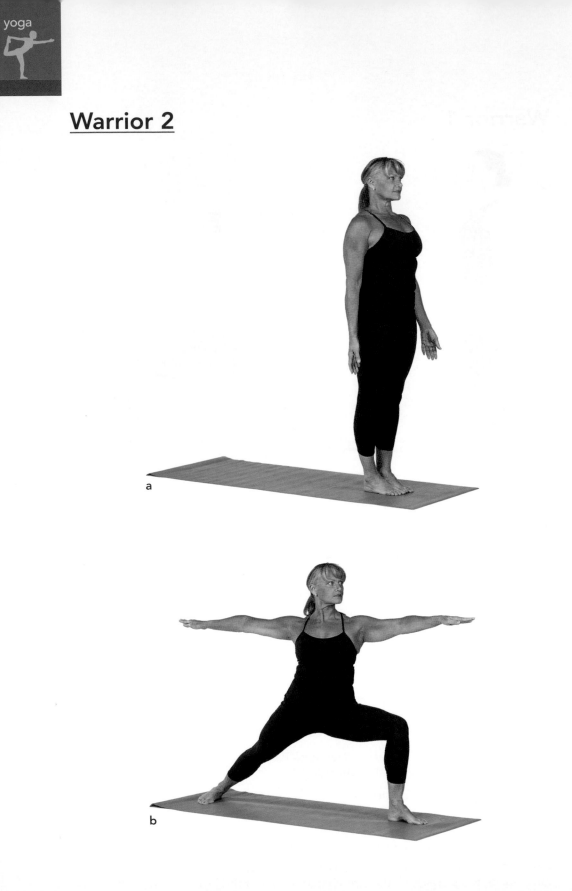

a

b

Starting Position Stand tall with the feet together or hip-width apart and the knees aligned directly over the center of the feet. Maintain a neutral spine. The shoulders are relaxed down and away from the ears and slightly back to open the front of the chest (see figure a).

Action Step one leg behind you and bend the front knee to just above 90 degrees, lined up directly over the ankle. Keep the back leg straight. Externally rotate the back hip to turn the toes out and open the hip to 90 degrees. Press the outside edge of the foot down while lifting the inner arch of the foot. Raise the arms to shoulder height, reaching one arm forward and the other back (see figure b). Look over the front hand. Keep the hip, knee, and foot of the front leg aligned. Roll the front hip under as you open the back hip. The arms reach without tension in the neck and shoulders.

Alignment Keep the front knee aligned over the center of the front foot. The shin forms a straight line from the knee to the heel. The ribs remain centered over the hips, and the pelvis is in a neutral alignment.

Breath Inhale to reach the arms out. Exhale to relax unwanted tension. Hold for three to five breaths per side.

Progressions and Modifications

- To increase the intensity of the exercise, lower the hips to form a 90-degree angle in the front knee.
- Stand higher in the lunge to decrease the intensity.

Mindfulness Bring your attention to your breath. Use the 3D breathing technique to give you strength in this challenging exercise. On the inhale, focus on strength. On the exhalation, release any unwanted tension. Find the balance between strength and calmness.

Reverse Warrior

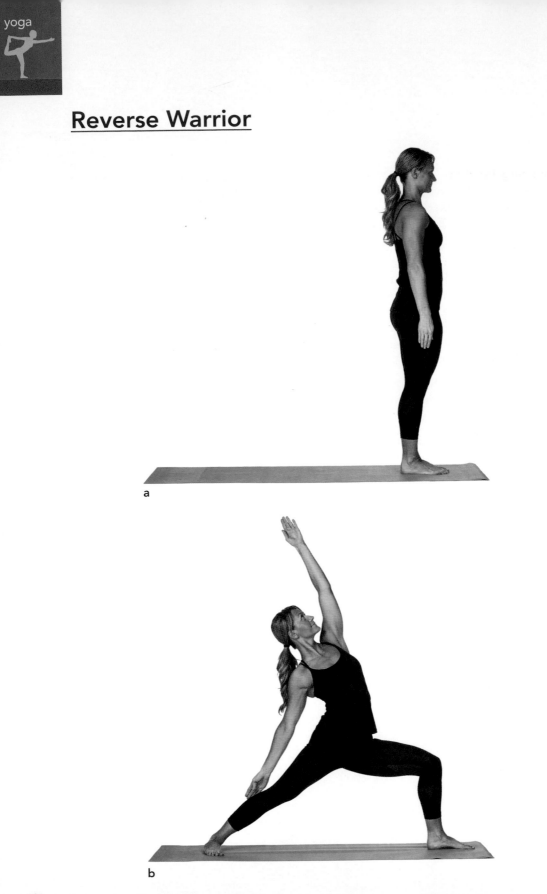

a

b

Starting Position   Stand tall with the feet together or hip-width apart and the knees aligned directly over the center of the feet. Maintain a neutral spine. The shoulders are relaxed and pulling down and away from the ears and slightly back to open the front of the chest (see figure *a*).

Action   Step one leg behind you and bend the front knee to just above 90 degrees, lined up directly over the ankle. Keep the back leg straight. Externally rotate the back hip to turn the toes out and open the hip to 90 degrees. Press the outside edge of the foot down while lifting the inner arch of the foot. Raise the arms to shoulder height, reaching one arm forward and the other back. Look over the front hand. Keep the hip, knee, and foot of the front leg aligned. Roll the front hip under as you open the back hip. Raise the front arm above your head, creating a stretch in the front of the waist as the opposite arm reaches toward the floor behind you (see figure *b*).

Alignment   Keep the front knee aligned over the center of the front foot. The shin forms a straight line from the knee to the heel. The ribs remain centered over the hips and the pelvis in a neutral alignment.

Breath   Inhale to reach the arm up. Exhale to relax unwanted tension. Hold for three to five breaths per side.

Progressions and Modifications
- To increase the intensity of the exercise, lower the hips to form a 90-degree angle in the front knee.
- Place the back hand on the thigh to support the back.
- Stand higher in the lunge to decrease the intensity.
- Fluidly move between warrior 2 and reverse warrior.

Mindfulness   Notice how you create space in the front of the torso by lifting the rib cage up and away from the hips without compressing the low back.

Extended Side Angle

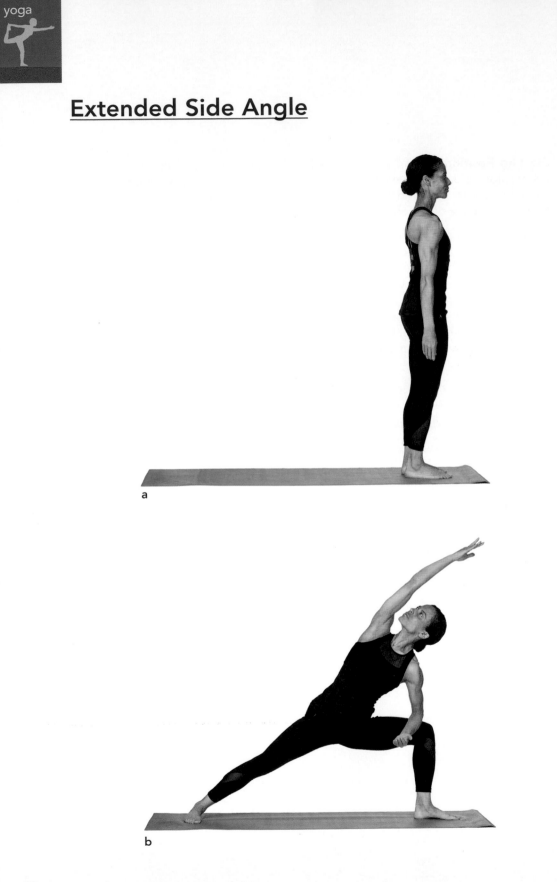

a

b

Starting Position   Stand tall with the feet together or hip-width apart and the knees aligned directly over the center of the feet. Maintain a neutral alignment of the spine. The shoulders are relaxed down and away from the ears and slightly back to open the front of the chest (see figure a).

Action   Step one leg behind you and bend the front knee to just above 90 degrees, lined up directly over the ankle. Open the back hip by externally rotating it and rolling the front hip under to turn the toes out and open the hip to 90 degrees. Press the outside edge of the foot down while lifting the inner arch of the foot. Raise the arms to shoulder height, reaching one arm forward and the other back. Slide the rib cage forward and bring the front forearm to the front thigh while reaching the back arm diagonally overhead, creating a diagonal line from the outer edge of the foot through the legs, torso, arm, and finally the fingertips (see figure b). Avoid collapsing the upper body into the front leg by keeping the waist lengthened and the core engaged. Look up toward the upper arm.

Alignment   Keep the hip, knee, and foot of the front leg aligned. Roll the front hip under as you open the back hip. Reach the arm overhead without tension in the shoulders. Avoid collapsing the upper body into the front leg by keeping the waist lengthened and the core engaged.

Breath   Inhale to reach forward as you begin the pose. Exhale to lower the front forearm to the thigh and reach the opposite arm overhead. Hold for three to five breaths per side.

Progressions and Modifications

- To increase intensity the exercise, lower the hips to form a 90-degree angle in the front knee.
- To increase the stretch, bring the front hand to the floor on the inside of the front foot.
- Stand higher in the lunge to decrease the intensity.
- Fluidly move between reverse warrior and extended side angle.

Mindfulness   Use the 3D breathing technique to engage the core and release unwanted tension.

Single-Leg Balance

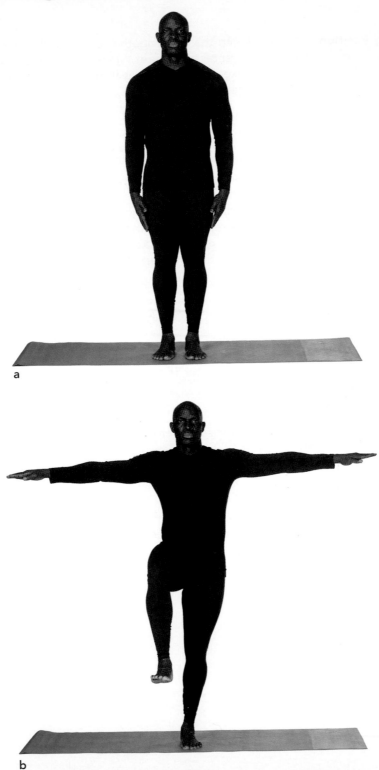

a

b

Starting Position   Stand tall with the feet together or shoulder-width apart, pressing equally into the four corners of the feet; contract the quadriceps muscles and feel as though you are pulling up toward the pelvis (see figure *a*). Lift from the pelvic floor and engage the abdominal muscles by drawing the belly button in and up toward the diaphragm. The chest is lifted and the gaze is straight ahead. The chin is slightly tucked to place the head in a neutral alignment.

Action   Bring the arms out to the side at shoulder height to assist with balance. Keep the spine in a neutral and lengthened position. Spread one foot firmly into the ground and lift the opposite leg to the front with the knee bent and the supporting leg straight (see figure *b*). Relax the shoulders down and away from the ears and slightly back to open the front of the chest.

Alignment   Focus your attention on creating a tall posture, lengthening from the feet to the top of the head. Keep the hips level and even with each other as you lift one leg.

Breath   Inhale to lift the leg into a balance. Breathe naturally to hold the single-leg balance for 5 to 10 breaths per side.

Technique Tips

- Press equally into the ball and heel of the foot.
- With the supporting leg straight, maintain the alignment of the knee over the foot.
- Keep the hips aligned with each other so that the pelvis remains level and you avoid tipping to one side.
- Relax the shoulders down and away from the ears and lift the chest.
- Keep your gaze soft.

Progressions and Modifications

- Hold the balance longer to increase intensity.
- Reach the arms overhead to challenge your balance.
- Bring the hands to the hips to bring awareness to pelvic alignment.
- Lower and lift the leg to add a dynamic challenge to the balance.
- To assist with balance, place your hands on the back of a chair or the wall.

Mindfulness   Focus your gaze on something that is still and quiet the mind to give you better balance. If the eyes wander, the mind will wander and the body will lose balance.

Side Balance

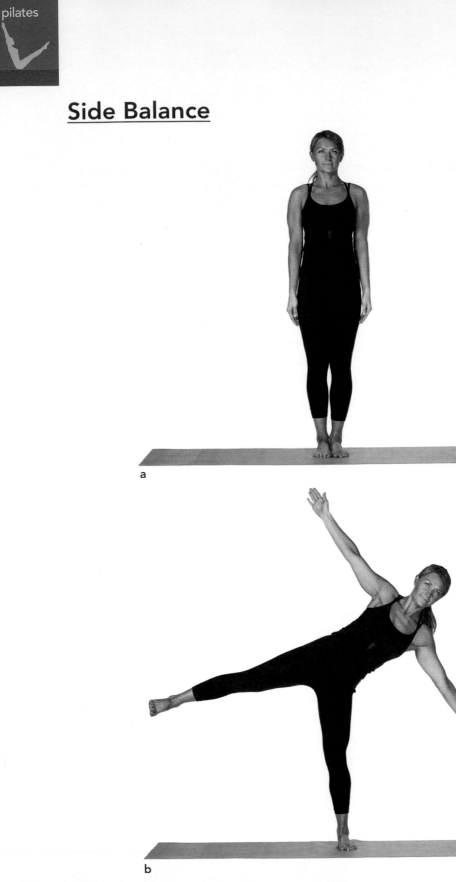

a

b

Starting Position   Stand tall with the feet together or shoulder-width apart, pressing equally into the four corners of the feet. Contract the quadriceps muscles and feel as though you are pulling up toward the pelvis (see figure a). Lift upward from the pelvic floor and engage the abdominal muscles by drawing the navel in and up toward the diaphragm. The chest is lifted and the gaze is straight ahead with a slight chin tuck to place the head in a neutral alignment. Focus your attention on creating a tall posture, lengthening from the feet to the top of the head.

Action   Keeping both legs straight, press one foot firmly into the ground and lift the other foot while tilting the body to the side over the supporting leg (see figure b). Reach the arms out to the side at shoulder height. Maintain this alignment as you tilt to the side.

Alignment   The supporting leg is straight, and the spine is in a neutral alignment. The shoulders relax down and away from the ears and slightly back to open the front of the chest. Maintain this alignment as you tilt to the side.

Breath   Inhale to lift the leg to a balance. Exhale to tilt to the side. Breathe naturally to hold the single-leg balance for three to five breaths per side.

Progressions and Modifications
  ▪ Hold the balance longer to increase intensity.
  ▪ Reach the arms overhead to challenge your balance.
  ▪ Lower and lift the leg to add a dynamic challenge to the balance and develop outer-hip strength.
  ▪ To assist with balance, place your hands on the back of a chair or the wall.

Mindfulness   Imagine you are standing between two panes of glass so the body moves neither forward nor back.

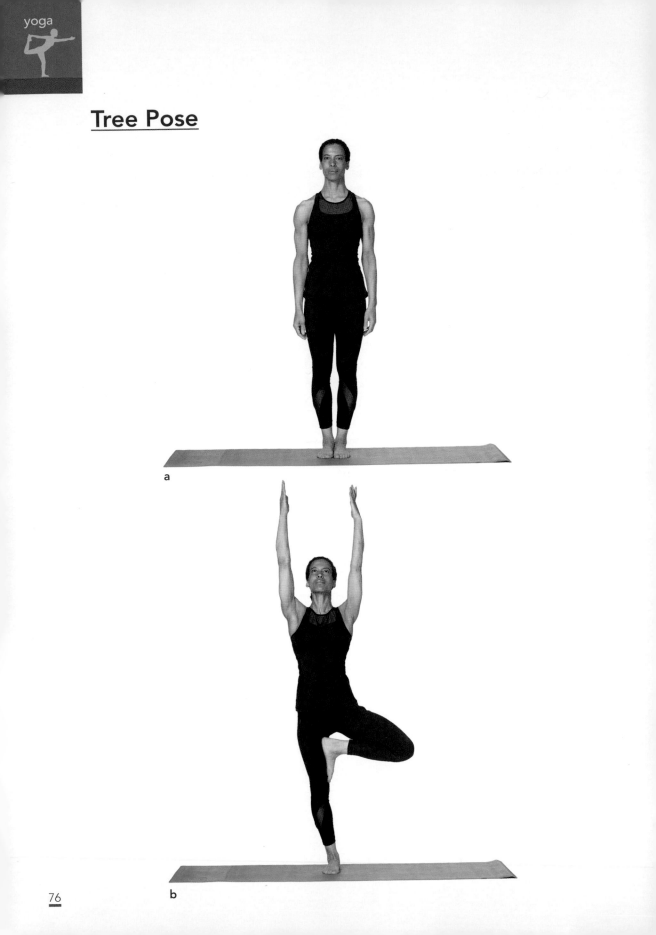

Tree Pose

a

b

Starting Position Stand tall with the feet together or shoulder-width apart. Pressing equally into the four corners of the feet, contract the quadriceps muscles and feel as though you are pulling up toward the pelvis. Lift upward from the pelvic floor and engage the abdominal muscles by drawing the belly button in and up toward the diaphragm. The chest is lifted, the gaze is straight ahead, the chin is tucked slightly to place the head in a neutral alignment, and the arms are down by your side. Focus your attention on creating a tall posture, lengthening from the feet to the top of the head (see figure *a*).

Action Press one foot firmly into the ground, keeping the leg straight, and lift the opposite foot. Open the hip to the side and place the sole of the other foot against the inside of the ankle, calf, or inner thigh of the supporting leg (see figure *b*). The shoulders relax down and away from the ears and slightly back to open the front of the chest. Keep the hips level and avoid rotating the hips and back as you lift the leg.

Alignment The supporting leg is straight and the spine is in a neutral alignment. The shoulders relax down and away from the ears and slightly back to open the front of the chest. Keep the hips level and avoid rotating the hips and back as you lift the leg into tree pose.

Breath Inhale to lift the leg to a balance. Exhale to open the hips and place the foot on the supporting leg. Breathe naturally to hold the single-leg balance for three to five breaths per side.

Progressions and Modifications

- Hold the balance longer to increase intensity.
- Reach the arms overhead to challenge your balance.
- To assist with balance, place your hands on the back of a chair or the wall.

Mindfulness Focus on the rhythm of the breath. With each exhalation, root the supporting foot more strongly into the ground. With each inhalation, create a sensation of lifting from the foot out through the crown of the head.

Warrior 3

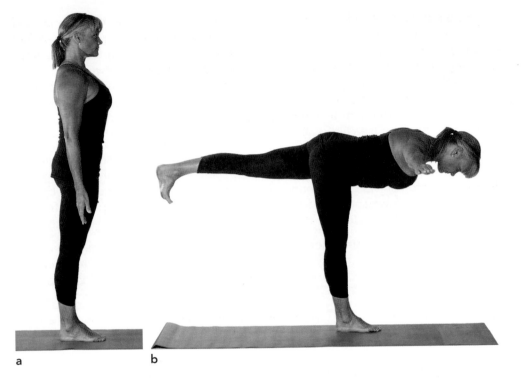

a b

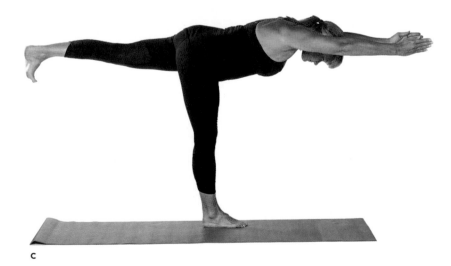

c

Starting Position   Stand tall with the feet together or shoulder-width apart, pressing equally into the four corners of the feet; contract the quadriceps muscles and feel as though you are pulling up toward the pelvis (see figure a). Lift upward from the pelvic floor and engage the abdominal muscles by drawing the navel in and up toward the diaphragm. The chest is lifted and the gaze is straight ahead, with a slight chin tuck to place the head in a neutral alignment and the arms down by your side. Focus your attention on creating a tall posture, lengthening from the feet to the top of the head.

Action   Lift the arms out to the sides at shoulder height. Shift your weight on to one leg and with that leg straight, lift the opposite leg back while tilting the torso forward. The torso, head, and lifted leg are in a straight line to form a T-shape with the body (see figure b).

Alignment   The supporting leg is straight, the spine is in a neutral alignment, and the head is in line with the back. The shoulders are relaxed down and away from the ears and slightly back to open the front of the chest. Tilt only as far forward as you can to maintain a straight line through the body from your head to the toe of the lifted leg. Keep the hips level and aligned with each other.

Breath   Exhale as you pivot from the hips to lift the leg and tilt the body. Breathe naturally to hold the single-leg balance for three to five breaths per side. Inhale to return to standing.

Progressions and Modifications
- Hold the balance longer to increase intensity.
- Change the arm position to reach the arms overhead to challenge your balance (see figure c).
- Position the arms overhead and move them in a swimming motion with one arm lifting and the other lowering to add a core challenge.
- Lower and lift the leg to add a dynamic challenge to the balance.
- To assist with balance, place your hands on the back of a chair or the wall.

Mindfulness   Quiet your mind of doubt and replace your thoughts with words of strength.

Half Moon

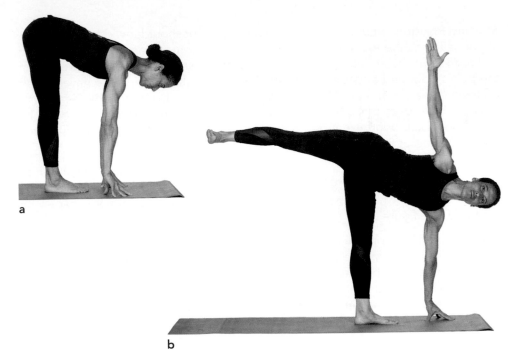

a

b

Starting Position From a standing position, hinge forward to assume a forward-bend position (see figure a). The spine is in a neutral alignment.

Action Place the fingertips of one hand approximately a torso length in front of one foot and keeping the leg straight, lift the opposite leg up until it is parallel with the floor, turning the hip open with the toe pointed to the side while maintaining a neutral spine (see figure b). Place your other hand on your hip or extend it up toward the ceiling while opening the chest. Keep the lifted leg active by gently flexing the ankle and pressing the heel back.

Alignment The supporting leg is straight, and the spine is in a neutral alignment. Open the front of the chest.

Breath Inhale to lift the leg into the balance. Exhale to extend through both legs. Breathe naturally to hold the single-leg balance for three to five breaths per side.

Progressions and Modifications
- Hold the balance longer to increase intensity.
- Lower and lift the leg to add a dynamic challenge to the balance.
- Look to the floor to assist with balance or look up to the extended arm to challenge balance.
- Place your hands on the back of a chair or a yoga block to help maintain balance and alignment.

Mindfulness Stand firm on your supporting leg and trust yourself.

6

Floor Strength, Balance, and Flexibility Exercises

The fusion floor exercises build strength, balance, and flexibility in the upper and lower body while integrating core training. The floor exercises define the muscles of the arms, legs, buttocks, back, and abdominals by focusing on proper alignment and posture.

The exercises in this section are grouped according to movement patterns and build from a foundational movement. As you learned in the previous chapter, a foundational movement uses a body position or exercise that is common in other exercises. For example, a plank is a foundational exercise for push-ups and many Pilates-based exercises. Once you learn the position, execution, and technique required in the foundational exercise, you can apply that information to the other exercises that use a similar movement pattern. Grouping the exercises this way makes it easy to move from one exercise to the next with minimal adjustments in body position during a fusion workout. Not only is this more efficient, but it also helps you master the exercise technique. A variety of exercise options are available from the foundational exercise. Using the fusion method, you will be able to easily mix and match the exercises within each group to flow from one exercise to another, to change the intensity, and to bring novelty to your workouts.

FOUNDATIONAL EXERCISE

Plank Position

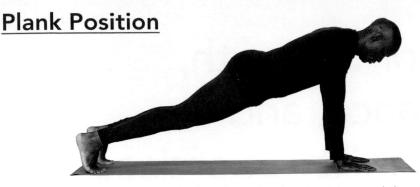

Starting Position   Kneel with the hands under the shoulders, stabilize the shoulders and contract the core muscles to extend one leg back, curling the toes under to balance on the ball of the foot with the heel aligned directly over the toes. Step the opposite leg back, keeping the core strong and the torso in a neutral alignment. The spine is in a neutral alignment with a slight lumbar curve and the hips in line with the spine. The head aligns with the spine. The arms are vertical under the shoulders, and the shoulder blades are drawn back and in with the chest open. Spread the hands into the floor, pointing the middle finger directly forward and the thumb reaching toward the center.

Action   Press into the hands to draw energy up the arms to the shoulder girdle. Widen the chest and bring the shoulder blades toward the midline of the back. Keep the upper body working and gently pull the deep abdominal muscles up toward the spine. Firm the muscles of the legs and lift the pelvic floor and lower-abdominal muscles to engage the deep core muscles (see figure).

Alignment   The spine maintains a neutral alignment, with the head in line with the spine, creating a straight line through the entire body.

Breath   To activate the muscles of the core, use the 3D breathing technique. Exhale to lift the abdominal muscles in and up while creating internal tension within the abdominals. Inhale to stay strong in the exercise. Hold for 5 to 15 breaths.

Technique Tips

- Slightly tuck the chin to draw the head back in line with the spine.
- Keep the arms in a vertical line and avoid rounding the upper back.
- Maintain the alignment of the spine, hips, and head.
- Avoid lifting the hips up or dropping the hips, creating an excessive curve in the low back.
- Spread the fingers wide to disperse the weight through the hand.
- Engage the muscles of the upper back and core to decrease the pressure on the wrists.
- Keep the muscles of the legs firm to support the weight of the pelvis.
- Lift the abdominal muscles toward the spine without changing the position of the spine.

Progressions and Modifications

- To decrease the intensity, bend the knees to bring them the floor.
- To decrease wrist discomfort, bring the forearms to the floor.

Mindfulness   Focus your attention on working the core muscles through the use of strong breath work to gain strength and endurance.

Plank With Leg Lift

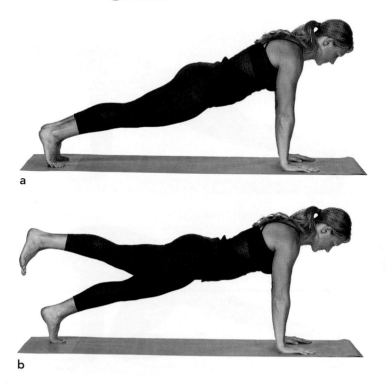

a

b

Starting Position   Assume a plank position. The spine is in a neutral alignment with a slight lumbar curve, and the hips and head are in line with the spine. The arms are vertical under the shoulders, and the shoulder blades are drawn back and in to open the chest. Spread the hands into the floor, pointing the middle finger directly forward with the thumb reaching toward the center (see figure a).

Action   Maintain perfect plank alignment and lift one leg straight up to hip height with a flexed ankle (see figure b). Point the toe then flex the ankle while the foot is lifted and lower to repeat on the other leg.

Alignment   The spine maintains a neutral alignment, with the head in line with the spine, creating a straight line through the body.

Breath   Inhale to lift the leg. Exhale to flex the ankle. Inhale to point the toe, and exhale to lower the foot. Repeat 5 to10 times per side.

Progressions and Modifications

▌ To add intensity, bend the knee to a 90-degree angle, keeping the inner thighs together. Inhale to curl the knee in, lift the knee on an exhalation, and lower the knee on an inhalation. Extend the leg out to plank and repeat on the other side.

▌ To decrease discomfort in the wrists, place the forearms on the floor.

Mindfulness   Imagine you are balancing a plate of glass on the back of the pelvis, and you want to keep it from falling as you move from one leg to the other.

Knee-Tuck Series

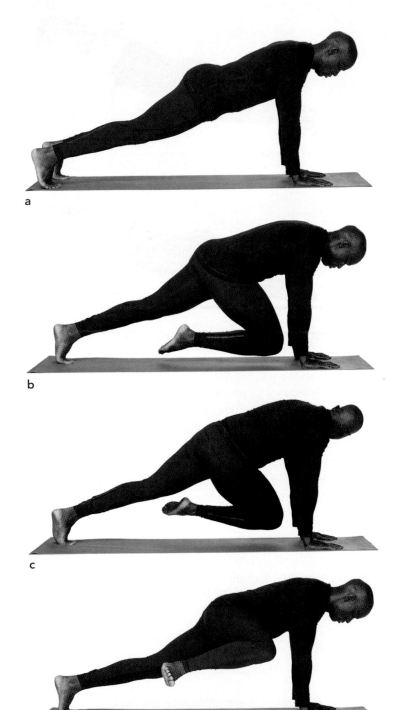

a

b

c

d

Starting Position   Assume a plank position. The spine is in a neutral alignment, with a slight lumbar curve and the hips and head are in line with the spine. The arms are vertical under the shoulders, and the shoulder blades are drawn back and in to open the chest. Spread the hands into the floor, pointing the middle finger directly forward and the thumb reaching toward the center (see figure a).

Action   While in the plank, lift one leg to hip height. Bend the knee and bring the knee toward the chest while keeping the spine in a neutral alignment (see figure b). Extend the leg back out to plank. Repeat and bring the knee to the opposite shoulder (see figure c) and return to plank. Finally, lift the leg and bring the knee to the elbow on the same side of the body (see figure d) and return to plank. Repeat the sequence with the other leg.

Alignment   In the plank position, the spine maintains a neutral alignment. The head is in line with the spine, creating a straight line through the body.

Breath   Inhale to lift the leg. Exhale to tuck the leg in. Inhale to return the leg to the start position. Perform one to six repetitions per side.

Progressions and Modifications

- To decrease intensity, lower the knees to the floor and come to a tabletop position in which you are on all fours. Bring one leg in to a tuck position and then extend it directly back as you lift the leg, straight and long.
- To decrease the intensity, perform one tuck at a time and take breaks between each variation of the exercise.
- To increase the challenge, keep the leg lifted between the three knee-tuck variations.

Mindfulness   This exercise requires determination. Believe in yourself and you will do this.

Plank With Hip Drive

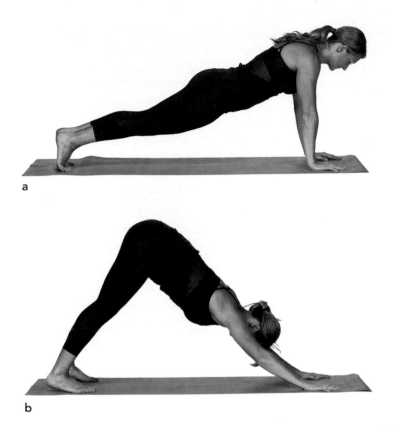

a

b

Starting Position Assume a plank position. The spine is in a neutral alignment with a slight lumbar curve, and the hips and head are in line with the spine. The arms are vertical under the shoulders, and the shoulder blades are drawn back and in to open the chest. Spread the hands into the floor, pointing the middle finger directly forward and the thumb reaching toward the center (see figure a).

Action From the plank position, drive the hips upward to a pike, keeping the heels lifted (see figure b). Keep the core engaged as you return to plank position.

Alignment In the plank position, the spine maintains a neutral alignment and the head is in line with the spine, creating a straight line through the body.

Breath Inhale to pike the hips upward. Exhale to lower to plank. Breathing should be strong, slow, and purposeful. Repeat 8 to 12 times.

Progressions and Modifications

- To add challenge, lift one arm up and swing it back toward the hips in the pike position and forward in the plank.
- To reduce wrist discomfort, perform the exercise from the forearms.

Mindfulness Create a flow between your breath and movement.

Plank to Hip Drop

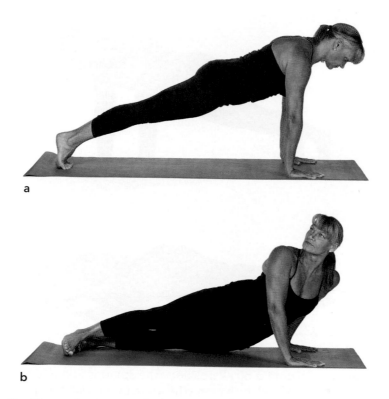

a

b

Starting Position Assume a plank position. The spine is in a neutral alignment with a slight lumbar curve, and the hips and head are in line with the spine. The arms are vertical under the shoulders, and the shoulder blades are drawn back and in to open the chest. Spread the hands into the floor, pointing the middle finger directly forward and the thumb reaching toward the center (see figure a).

Action From the plank position, lower one hip toward the floor (see figure b). Lift the hip to return to plank and repeat on the other side.

Alignment In the plank position, the spine maintains a neutral alignment. The head is in line with the spine, creating a straight line through the body.

Breath Exhale to lower the hip, inhale to lift the hip, and exhale to the other side. Repeat 5 to 10 times per side.

Progressions and Modifications
- To decrease intensity, lower the knees to the floor.
- To add intensity, increase the range of motion of the exercise by lifting the hips higher and lowering the hips to touch the floor.
- To decrease discomfort in the wrists, place the forearms on the floor.

Mindfulness Allow your body to move through a comfortable range of motion. Increase your range as you gain confidence and strength.

Narrow Push-Up

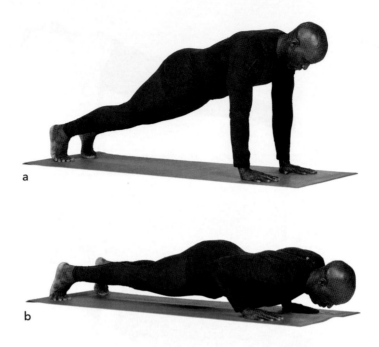

a

b

Starting Position Assume a plank position. The spine is in a neutral alignment with a slight lumbar curve, and the hips and head are in line with the spine. The arms are vertical under the shoulders, and the shoulder blades are drawn back and in to open the chest. Spread the hands into the floor, pointing the middle finger directly forward and the thumb reaching toward the center (see figure a).

Action From the plank position, shift the body weight forward onto the arms and hug the upper arms into the side of the ribs to lower into a push-up (see figure b). Keep the core working as you lower your body. Push down through the hands and press back up to plank.

Alignment The spine maintains a neutral alignment. The head is in line with the spine, creating a straight line through the body.

Breath Inhale and exhale to set the core using a fusion 3D breath. Inhale to lower into the push-up, and exhale to return to the start. Complete 5 to 10 repetitions.

Progressions and Modifications
- To decrease the intensity, lower the knees to the floor.
- Lower to the depth you can hold ideal alignment. To increase intensity, go lower into the push-up.
- To add intensity, lift one leg.

Mindfulness Focus on being strong. In your mind, celebrate your personal strength.

Wide Push-Up

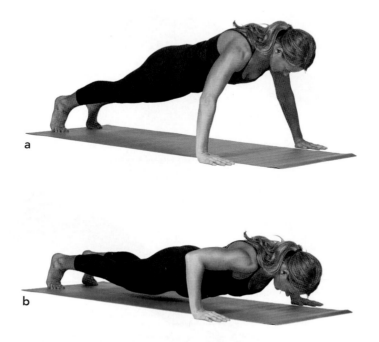

a

b

Starting Position   Assume a plank position. The spine is in a neutral alignment with a slight lumbar curve, and the hips and head are in line with the spine (see figure *a*). Place the hands wider than shoulder-width apart. The shoulder blades are drawn back and in to open the chest. Spread the hands into the floor.

Action   Slightly rotate the fingers inward to comfortably allow the elbows to bend outward as you lower into the push-up (see figure *b*). Keeping the core muscles engaged, press down into the hands to return to the start position, maintaining neutral alignment of the spine.

Alignment   The spine maintains a neutral alignment. The head is in line with the spine, creating a straight line through the body.

Breath   Inhale and exhale to set the core using a fusion 3D breath. Inhale to lower in the push-up, and exhale to return to the start. Complete 5 to 10 repetitions.

Progressions and Modifications

- To decrease the intensity, lower the knees to the floor.
- Lower to the depth you can hold ideal alignment. As you progress go lower into the push-up.
- To add intensity, lift one leg.

Mindfulness   Focus on your breath to give you strength.

Side Plank

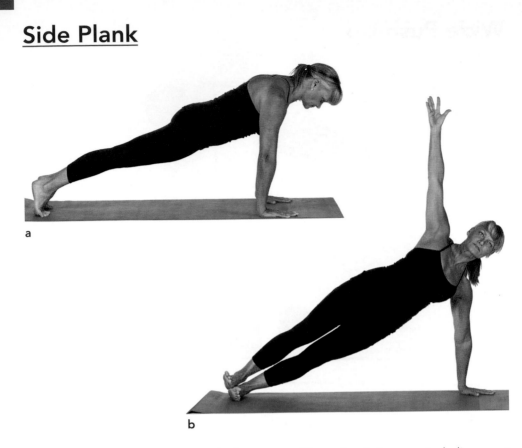

a

b

Starting Position   Assume a plank position. The spine is in a neutral alignment with a slight lumbar curve, and the hips and head are in line with the spine. The arms are vertical under the shoulders, with the shoulder blades drawn back and in to open the chest. Spread the hands into the floor, pointing the middle finger directly forward and the thumb reaching toward the center (see figure a).

Action   From the plank position, bring one hand in line with the center of the chest. Open the body to the side as you lift the opposite arm to reach toward the ceiling (see figure b).

Alignment   The body creates a long line from head to toe.

Breath   Inhale to set the hand and engage the core. Exhale to rotate into the side plank. Breathe deeply to hold the position for three to five breaths per side.

Progressions and Modifications

- To decrease discomfort in the wrists, place the forearms on the floor.
- To add a balance challenge, stack the feet on top of each other.
- To add a strength challenge, lift the top leg to hip height.
- To decrease the intensity, lower the bottom knee to the floor to a bent-knee position.

Mindfulness   Imagine that your body is between two panes of glass.

FOUNDATIONAL EXERCISE

Tabletop

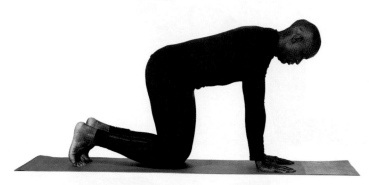

Starting Position   Assume a kneeling position, place the hands directly under the shoulders, and spread the fingers spread wide. The knees are directly under the hips, creating a vertical line with the thighs. The spine and pelvis are in a neutral alignment from head to hips.

Action   Stabilize the shoulder girdle and contract the core muscles to brace the spine and maintain neutral spinal alignment. Avoid tucking the pelvis under. Press the shoulders down and away from the ears and slightly back to open the front of the chest (see figure).

Alignment   Align the head with the spine and slightly tuck the chin to point the crown of the head forward.

Breath   Inhale to set the hands and knee position. Exhale to engage the core muscles to brace the spine in this position. Hold for three to five breaths.

Technique Tips

- Spread the hands wide for a better base of support.
- Keep the arms straight and move the shoulder blades toward the middle of the back.
- Lift the navel upward toward the spine by engaging the deep inner-core muscles.
- Maintain the alignment of the knees with the feet and keep the knees from falling inward or outward.

Progressions and Modifications

- To increase the intensity, lift the knees a few inches off the floor.
- Place a rolled mat under the knees for comfort.

Mindfulness   This position creates a balanced and stable foundation for more challenging exercises. Focus on how the muscles of the core work three dimensionally and how different exercises work the core differently to achieve the movement.

Two-Point Tabletop

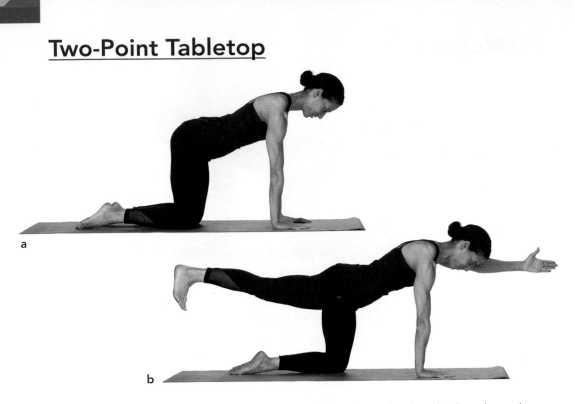

a

b

Starting Position   Assume a kneeling position, place the hands directly under the shoulders, and spread the fingers wide. The knees are directly under the hips, creating a vertical line with the thighs (see figure a). The spine and pelvis are in a neutral alignment from head to hips.

Action   From the tabletop position, lift one arm and reach it directly out in front. Lift the opposite leg and reach it directly back in the opposing direction (see figure b). The body should remain centered as the leg and arm lift.

Alignment   Keep the spine in a neutral alignment and avoid rolling the hips to one side. The lifted arm and leg should make a straight line from the heel of the foot to the finger tips.

Breath   Inhale to set the core muscles. Exhale to reach the arm and leg out. Hold for three to five breaths per side.

Progressions and Modifications

- To challenge the core differently, move the lifted arm and leg to the side at a diagonal.
- To decrease the intensity, lift only the arm or the leg at one time.
- To add variety and increase intensity, bend the knee of the lifted leg and bring it under you as you bring the opposite elbow in to touch the knee to the elbow.
- To focus on the hip and legs, lift one leg and cross it over the supporting leg to touch the toes to the floor. Arch the leg up and over and touch out to the side without rotating the spine and losing alignment.

Mindfulness   Focus internally to sense how the inner core is working to maintain stability against the forces of gravity.

FOUNDATIONAL EXERCISE

Front-Lying Position

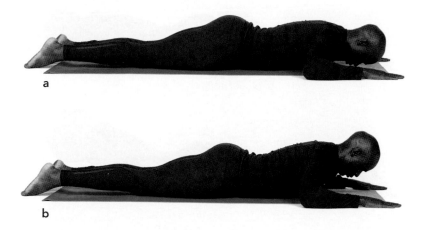

a

b

Starting Position   Lie in a prone position with the chest on the floor and the legs extended straight out from the hips and the tops of the feet on the floor so that the body creates a straight line from the head to the toes. Place the forearms comfortably on the floor with the palms of the hands facing down (see figure a).

Action   Contract the muscles of the legs to lift the knees off the floor and reach the legs out long from the hips. Lift the navel upward to the spine by engaging the deep abdominal muscles while pressing the pubic bone gently into the floor. Tuck the chin slightly and lift the head to align the head with the upper back. The tip of the nose points toward the floor (see figure b).

Alignment   The spine maintains a neutral alignment, with the head in line with the spine, creating a straight line through the body.

Breath   Inhale to lift the knees, and exhale to lift the abdominal muscles. Breathe naturally and hold for three to five breaths.

Technique Tips

▪ Press down lightly onto the tops of the feet in the start position.
▪ Keep the lifted sensation in the abdominal wall as you move into more advanced exercises.

Progressions and Modifications

▪ Place a towel under the forehead if it is difficult to maintain a neutral head alignment in the start position.
▪ To increase the intensity, place your hands on top of each other under the forehead in the start position.

Mindfulness   In this position, you will strengthen all of the muscles along the posterior (back) line of the body. Commonly, the gluteals and upper back muscles are weak causing the work to shift to the low back. Focus on keeping the abdominal muscles engaged to stabilize the low back.

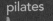
Back Extension

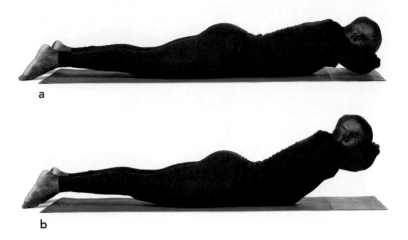

a

b

Starting Position   Begin in the front-lying position with the hands to the forehead (see figure *a*).

Action   Pull the navel up and in toward the spine and extend the upper back to lift the chest off the floor (see figure *b*). Press the tops of the feet into the floor as you lift up. Keep the abdominal muscles lifted to support the back.

Alignment   Keep the head in a neutral alignment with the upper back. Think of creating length rather than height.

Breath   Exhale to draw the abdominal muscles in. Inhale to lift the upper body. Exhale to lower. Repeat five to eight times.

Progressions and Modifications
■ Hold the top of the extension for a few breaths before lowering.
■ Reach the arms out straight to challenge strength.
■ Place the forearms on the floor to support the back extension.

Mindfulness   Imagine you are creating a gentle continuous curve from the head to the hips.

Swimmer

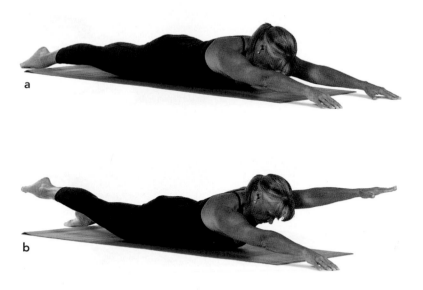

a

b

Starting Position Begin in the front-lying position. The arms are extended overhead, about shoulder-width apart and the palms down (see figure a).

Action Lift the upper body to a back extension and the legs in a low hip extension. Raise one arm and the opposing leg (see figure b). Switch and lift the other arm and leg while keeping the hips and low back stable. Move from one side to the other in a swimming motion.

Alignment Create length through the body by extending the top of the head and the feet in opposite directions. Keep the abdominal muscles lifted toward the spine.

Breath Inhale to raise one arm and the opposite leg. Exhale to switch. Continue the movement from side to side for 6 to 12 repetitions per side.

Progressions and Modifications

- To focus on the upper back and upper core strength, perform the arm actions only.
- To focus on lower body and lower core strength, perform the leg actions only.
- Vary the tempo of the movement to challenge core stability

Mindfulness Bring awareness to the core by pressing the front of the hips into the mat to maintain stability against the movement of the arms and legs.

Breaststroke

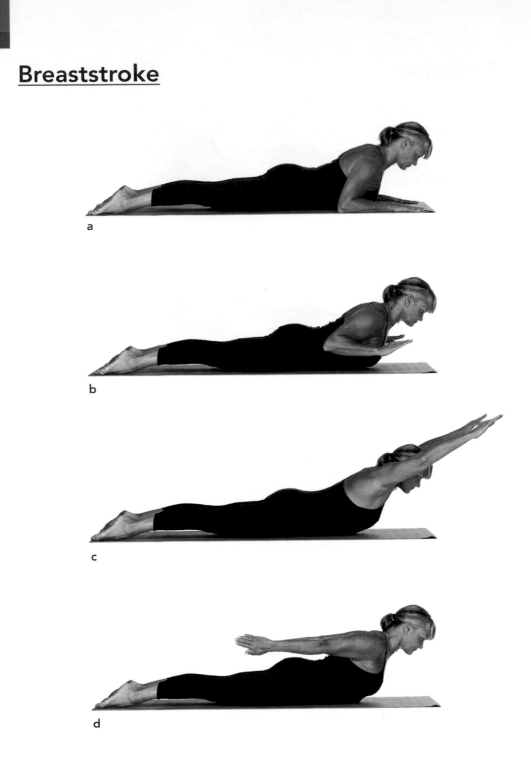

a

b

c

d

Starting Position   Begin in the front-lying position, with the tops of the feet pressed into the floor. Place the forearms on the floor beside the chest and ribs (see figure a). Extend the upper back into a low back extension and lift the hands off the floor by the shoulders (see figure b).

Action   Set the core by lifting the abdominal muscles. Keep the legs muscles active with the knees lifted off the floor and feet pressed down. Reach the arms forward with the palms facing down. (see figure c). Then pull the arms down to the side of the body as you lift higher in the upper back and open the front of the chest (see figure d). Return to the starting position.

Alignment   Create length through the body by extending the top of the head and the feet in opposite directions. Keep the abdominal muscles lifted toward the spine.

Breath   Inhale to lift the chest up. Exhale to reach the arms out straight in front. Inhale to pull the arms back to the side of the body. Exhale to return to the low back extension. Repeat 5 to 10 times.

Progressions and Modifications

- Vary the tempo by slowing the movement or increasing the speed.
- To decrease the intensity, rest between each repetition.

Mindfulness   Imagine that you are swimming and create the same fluidity with your movement and breath.

Hip Extension

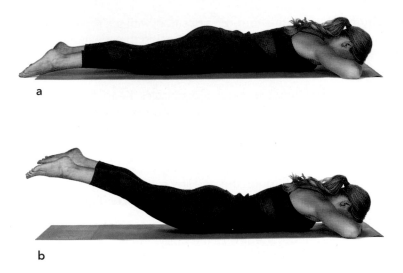

a

b

Starting Position   Begin in the front-lying position with the hands under the forehead and the legs approximately hip or shoulder width apart in a parallel rotated position (see figure a).

Action   Keeping the upper body in contact with the floor, lift the legs from the hips with the legs straight (see figure b). Think of lengthening the legs from the hips to lower them to the start position.

Alignment   Create length through the body by extending the top of the head and the feet in opposite directions. Lift the abdominal muscles toward the spine without putting tension on the neck and shoulders. Support the head in a neutral position.

Breath   Exhale to set the core muscles. Inhale to lift the legs. Exhale to lower. Repeat five to eight times.

Progressions and Modifications

- For variation and to change how the core works, lift one leg at a time.
- To add intensity, bend the knees to bring the heels to the hips and straighten keeping the fronts of the legs off the floor. Repeat the bend-and-straightening movement for several repetitions before resting.

Mindfulness   Focus on lifting the abdominal muscles to create a sensation of space in the low back.

Dynamic Bow

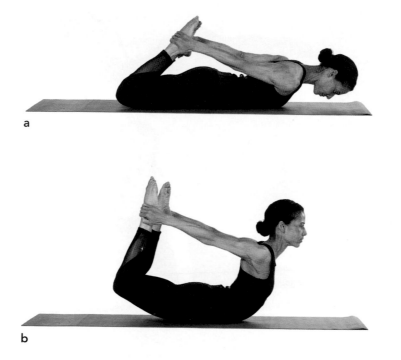

a

b

Starting Position   Begin in a front-lying position, with the knees bent and arms reaching behind to take hold of the outside of the ankles (see figure a).

Action   Lift the thighs off the floor by contracting the gluteal muscles and hamstrings. Press the feet into the hands and the shins back to lift the chest off the floor (see figure b).

Alignment   Keep the hands on the ankles as you lower to the start position. Create length through the upper body by extending the top of the head forward as you open the shoulders and chest to reach the arms back for the ankles. Lift the abdominal muscles toward the spine to support the low back.

Breath   Inhale to lift up into the bow. Hold the bow for 2 to 4 seconds. Exhale to lower. Repeat three to five times.

Progressions and Modifications

- To make the exercise easier, perform a half-bow exercise by lifting one arm and leg on the same side. Repeat on the other side.
- Lift one leg and reach back with the hand to the ankle, alternating each side dynamically in a controlled tempo.

Mindfulness   Use the legs to lift the chest and allow the low back to relax in the pose.

Upward-Facing Dog

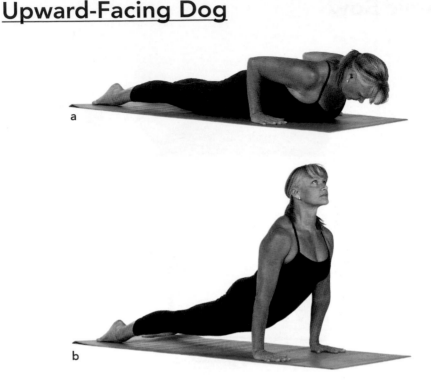

a

b

Starting Position Begin in a front-lying position with the hands beside the rib cage and the elbows pulled in and lifted up (see figure *a*).

Action Contract the muscles of the legs to lift the knees off the floor. Keeping the legs active, lift the chest into an upper-back extension. Maintain the extension in your back as you press into the hands and straighten the arms to lift the body and legs off the floor (see figure *b*).

Alignment Create length through the body by extending the top of the head and the feet in opposite directions. Lift the abdominal muscles toward the spine and firm the legs. The body should create a gentle extension from the head to the hips. The arms are in a vertical line from the shoulder to the wrist.

Breath Inhale to lift into upward-facing dog. Hold for one to five breaths. Exhale to lower to the start position.

Progressions and Modifications

- Keep the hips and legs on the floor and lift the chest in a low-back extension to decrease intensity.
- To make it easier, place the forearms on the floor and lift the chest for less spine extension.
- To take pressure off of the low back, curl the toes under and perform the exercise from the balls of the feet.

Mindfulness Imagine the sensation of opening your chest as if you are lifting your heart forward in this powerful yoga posture.

Seated Position

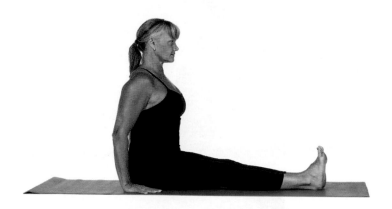

Starting Position   Sit on the center of the sitting bones. The legs are straight out in front and the torso is upright. The pelvis is neutral, with the rib cage over the hips and the head balanced over the spine, which is in neutral alignment.

Action   Place the hands on the floor beside the hips and gently press the hands down to lift through the spine. Lift the pelvic floor, bringing the navel inward and upward toward the spine (see figure). Open the chest and draw the shoulder blades back. Tuck the chin slightly and reach the crown of the head upward. Contract the quadriceps muscles and press the back of the legs down.

Alignment   Create a tall posture and long line from the sitting bones to the crown of the head.

Breath   Exhale to gently contract the inner-core muscles and stabilize a tall seated position. Breathe naturally for five breaths.

Technique Tips

- Press the legs down to create a sensation of lifting upward.
- Keep the lifted sensation of the abdominal wall as you move into more advanced exercises.

Progressions and Modifications

- Sit on a rolled yoga mat or yoga block to move the pelvis into a neutral alignment.
- Bend the knees if the hamstrings or low back are tight or in discomfort.

Mindfulness   This body position works the postural muscles of the core in a seated position. Be aware of the subtleness of the inner core working to bring you into a tall seated posture. Notice how your breath feels when you sit tall versus sinking into slouched posture.

Half Rollback

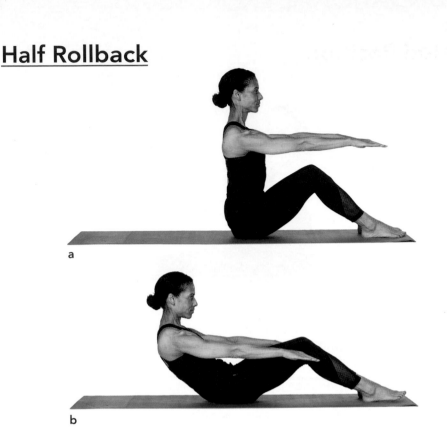

a

b

Starting Position   Begin in a tall seated position, with the knees bent and the feet on the floor about hip-width apart. Reach the arms out in front of the shoulders, with the palms of the hands facing down (see figure *a*). Relax the shoulders down and away from the ears.

Action   Roll back by rotating the pelvis under, contracting the abdominal muscles inward and the front of the rib cage downward. Slightly tuck the chin, leaving a fist distance between the chin and the chest and create a gentle curve through the spine from the pelvis to the middle of the back on the rollback. Continue to roll back until the low back just touches the floor (see figure *b*). To come up, begin by pulling the front of the rib cage down and curling up to a tall seated position.

Alignment   The spine is in a gentle curve from the hips to the head. Avoid tucking the chin too tightly or lifting the shoulders to the ears.

Breath   Inhale to sit tall. Exhale to roll back. Inhale and hold. Exhale to roll up to a tall seated position. Repeat 6 to 12 times.

Progressions and Modifications

- Place the hands behind the thighs to support the rollback and assist the curl-up to seated.
- For the oblique rollback, sweep one arm back, turning the palm of the hand up, slightly rotating to the side and looking toward the hand. Roll up and repeat on the other side.

Mindfulness   Focus on the movement of the pelvis and the spine as it flexes and extends without creating tension in the shoulders and neck.

Full Roll-Up

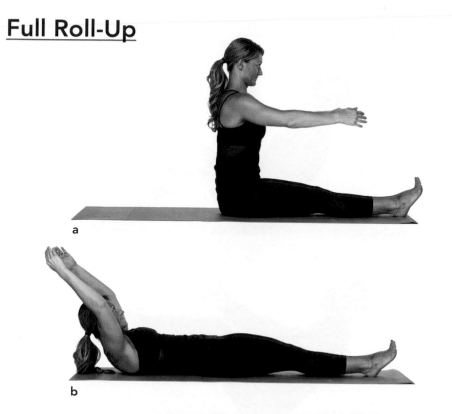

a

b

Starting Position Begin in a tall seated position, with the legs straight and the arms reaching out in front of the shoulders and the palms facing toward each other (see figure *a*). Relax the shoulders down and away from the ears.

Action Roll back by rotating the pelvis under, contracting the abdominal muscles inward and the front of the rib cage downward. Slightly tuck the chin, leaving a fist width between the chin and the chest and create a gentle curve through the spine from the pelvis to the middle of the back on the rollback. Continue to roll back, placing the back of the torso gently on the floor and reaching the arms overhead (see figure *b*). To come up, reach the arms over the chest, tuck the chin, and pull the front of the rib cage down. Continue to move the ribs to the hips to roll up to a tall seated position.

Alignment Begin the curve of the spine from the hips to the head as you roll back. On the roll-up, begin by tucking the chin and rolling from the upper back to the hips.

Breath Inhale to sit tall. Exhale to roll back. Inhale to reach the arms over the chest. Exhale to roll up to a tall seated position. Repeat four to eight times.

Progressions and Modifications

- Bend the knees and place the hands behind the thighs to support the rollback and assist in the curl-up to the seated position.
- For variation and to change how the core muscles work, circle the arms out to the side and overhead as you roll back.

Mindfulness Imagine the legs are anchored to the floor to allow the torso to roll through this movement.

V-Sit

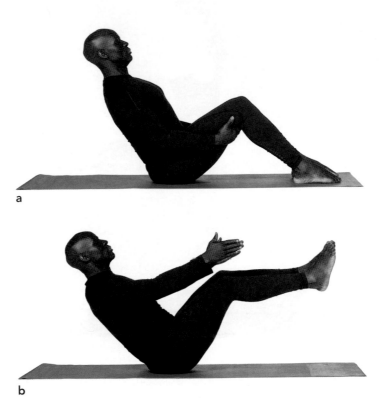

a

b

Starting Position   Begin in a tall seated position, with the knees bent and the hands behind the thighs (see figure *a*).

Action   Lean back to balance on the back of your sitting bones, keeping the back straight and forming a V-shape. Lift the feet off the floor and remove the hands from behind the legs to reach straight out from the shoulders (see figure *b*).

Alignment   Maintain a straight back. Avoid letting the hips roll back.

Breath   Inhale to sit tall. Exhale to lean back. Inhale and hold. Hold for four to eight breaths.

Progressions and Modifications
- Place the hands behind the thighs to support the back.
- To increase the challenge, reach the arms to the ceiling.
- To advance the exercise, straighten the legs.
- For variation and to challenge the core differently, in a straight-leg position cross the legs.
- Bring the forearms to the floor to support the back.

Mindfulness   Lift the chest as if the sternum were being pulled up by a string.

Reverse Table

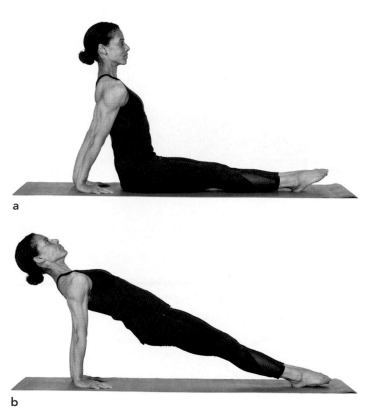

a

b

Starting Position Begin in a tall seated position with the hands on the floor approximately 6 inches (15 cm) behind you and the fingers turned toward the hips (see figure *a*).

Action Firm the legs and bring the inner thighs together. Press down into the hands and lift the hips and legs, creating a reverse plank position from head to toe (see figure *b*). The arms are vertical under the shoulders.

Alignment The body creates a long line from the feet to the shoulders. Tuck the chin slightly to support the weight of your head. The arms are in a vertical line in the lifted reverse-plank position.

Breath Inhale to sit tall. Exhale to lift into the plank. Inhale and hold. Exhale to lower. Repeat 6 to 10 times.

Progressions and Modifications

- To decrease the intensity, bend the knees and form a tabletop.
- To increase flexibility in the front of the shoulder and chest, keep the hips on the floor and practice the arm movement.

Mindfulness Be patient with yourself. Through practice and determination, this exercise will get easier.

FOUNDATIONAL EXERCISE

Side-Lying Position

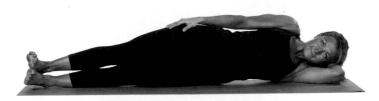

Starting Position   Lie on your side with your head, ribs, spine, and hips in a neutral position and the legs straight. Support your head with the lower arm and place the other hand on the floor in front of the chest to support you.

Action   Lift the waist off the floor to align the ribs and hips on top of each other (see figure). This will work the muscles of the front, side, and back of the core.

Alignment   The spine is in a neutral position, and the hips and ribs are stacked directly on top of each other.

Breath   Exhale to contract the muscles of the core and lift the waist. Breathe naturally for five breaths.

Technique Tips
- Slide the rib cage toward the bottom hip.
- Support the head by placing it on the bottom arm or a rolled towel to prevent neck fatigue.

Progressions and Modifications
- Bend the knees to decrease discomfort in the hips.
- Bend the bottom knee and keep the top leg straight to decrease intensity.

Mindfulness   This body position works the core muscles that support the low back. In doing the exercises in this position, focus your attention on the muscles along the side of the torso from the hips to shoulders and on how they work in unison to create stability and movement.

Side Leg Lift

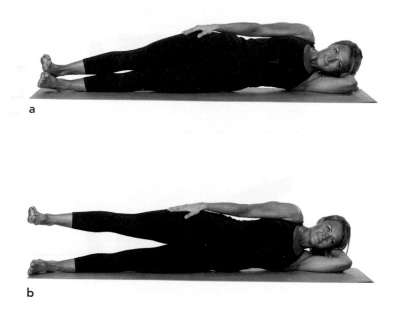

a

b

Starting Position   Begin in a side-lying position (see figure a).

Action   Keeping the waist lifted and the body in a straight line, lift the top leg slightly higher than hip height (see figure b).

Alignment   With the body in a straight line from head to toe, roll back slightly as you lift the leg to take pressure off the bones of the bottom of the hip.

Breath   Inhale to lift the leg. Exhale to lower the leg. Repeat 8 to 12 times per side.

Progressions and Modifications

- To increase the intensity, lift both legs.
- Bend the bottom knee for comfort.

Mindfulness   Let the movement occur without great force. Be soft and strong.

Side Leg Circle

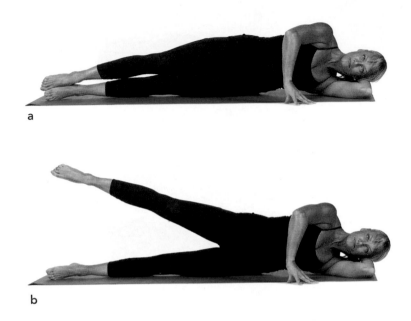

a

b

Starting Position   Begin in a side-lying position (see figure a).

Action   Lift the top leg to hip height and circle the leg in one direction without moving the hip or torso and keeping the body in a straight line (see figure b). Repeat the circle in the opposite direction. Repeat this sequence with the other leg.

Alignment   With the body in a straight line from head to toe, roll back slightly as you lift the legs to take pressure off of the hip.

Breath   Lift one leg; inhale on the first half of the circle. Exhale on the second half of the circle. Repeat 10 times in both directions per side.

Progressions and Modifications

  ❚ To increase the challenge, bring yourself to a side plank on your forearm.
  ❚ For the most advanced options, bring yourself to a side plank on your hand.

Mindfulness   Imagine drawing a perfect circle in the air with the toes.

Side Bend

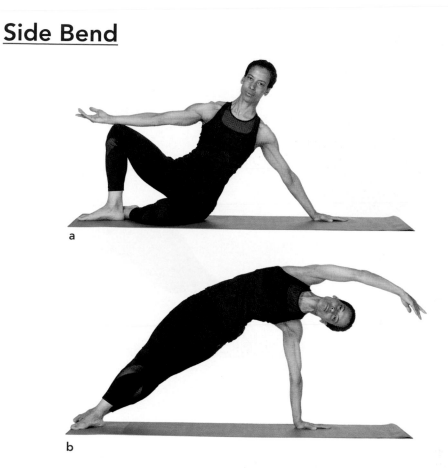

a

b

Starting Position   Begin in a seated position with the ankles crossed and the top knee pointed to the ceiling. Place one hand on the floor with the fingers pointed out and the arm straight at a slight angle forward from the shoulder. The other hand is placed with the palm facing up and the wrist extended across the top knee (see figure a).

Action   Lift from the bottom hip to laterally flex over the supporting arm and reach the opposite arm overhead in an arch as the legs straighten and squeeze together creating a side bend with the body (see figure b). Lower to the start position.

Alignment   At the top of the side bend, the supporting arm is vertical and the body creates an arch with the bottom hip and waist lifted. The hips and ribs are stacked on top of each other.

Breath   Inhale to initiate the lift. Exhale to finish the side bend. Inhale to hold the side bend. Exhale to lower to the start position. Repeat three to five times per side.

Progressions and Modifications

▪ To decrease intensity, keep the bottom knee bent on the floor.
▪ To decrease wrist discomfort, place the forearm on the floor.

Mindfulness   Imagine the body movement as similar to the arching of water in a fountain.

Side Twist

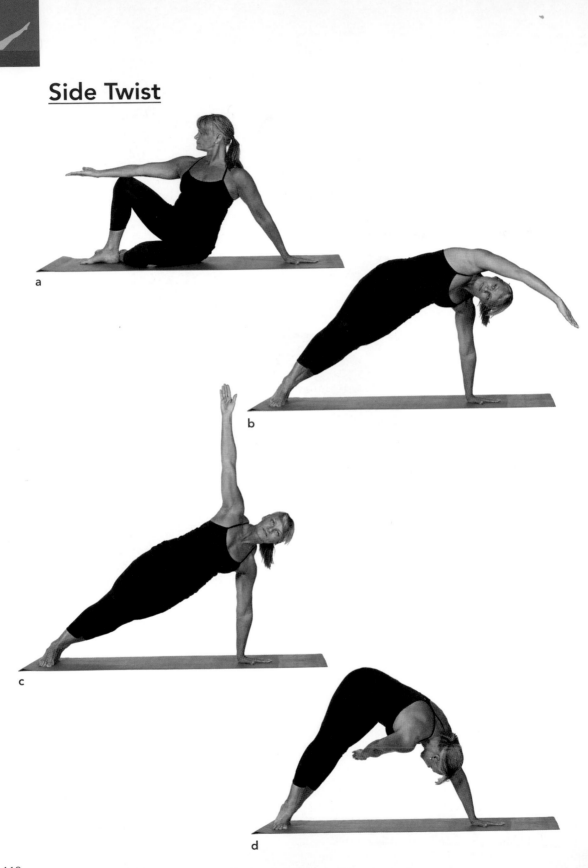

a

b

c

d

Starting Position   Begin in a seated position with the ankles crossed and the top knee pointed to the ceiling. Place one hand on the floor with the fingers pointed out and the arm straight at a slight angle forward from the shoulder. The other hand is placed with the palm facing up and the wrist extended across the top knee (see figure *a*).

Action   Lift from the bottom hip to laterally flex over the supporting arm and reach the opposite arm overhead in an arch as the legs straighten and squeeze together creating a side bend with the body (see figure *b*). Reach the top arm upward into a side plank (see figure *c*), then bend the elbow to reach the arm under the torso toward the opposite leg as you lift the hips into a pike (see figure *d*). The twist comes from the upper torso moving the rib cage toward the opposite hip. Return to the arm reaching up in a side plank. Lower to the starting position.

Alignment   At the top of the side bend, the supporting arm is vertical and the body creates an arch with the bottom hip lifted and the waist contracted. The hips and ribs are stacked on top of each other.

Breath   Inhale to initiate the lift. Exhale to finish the side bend. Inhale to reach the arm up. Exhale to twist and reach to the opposite hip. Inhale to reach up. Exhale to lower to the start position. Repeat three to five times per side.

Progressions and Modifications

- To decrease intensity, keep the bottom knee bent on the floor.
- To decrease wrist discomfort, place the forearms on the floor.

Mindfulness   Create a flow between breath and movement.

Abdominal Brace Position

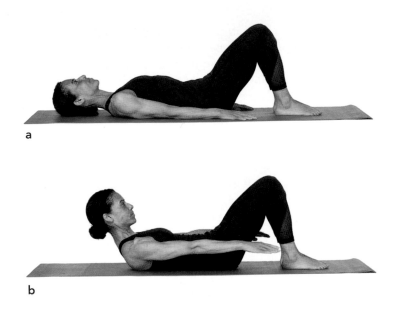

a

b

Starting Position   Lie on your back. The spine and pelvis are in a neutral alignment, the knees bent, and the feet on the floor and in line with the sitting bones. Place your arms on the floor at the side of the body, palms down (see figure a).

Action   Lengthen the back of the neck and bring the shoulder blades against the back of the rib cage. Keep the shoulder blades down as you flex the thoracic spine by moving the front of the rib cage toward the pelvis, reaching the arms out. Draw the navel toward the spine as you contract the deep inner-core muscles (see figure b).

Alignment   The hips are anchored to the floor as the ribs move toward the hips and the shoulders lift slightly off the floor.

Breath   Inhale to prepare. Exhale to contract the muscles of the core to slide the front of the ribs to the hips. Inhale and hold. Exhale to lower. Repeat 5 to 10 times.

Technique Tips
 ▮ Slide the bottom of the rib cage toward the hips.
 ▮ Slightly tuck the chin.

Progressions and Modifications
 ▮ To practice the action of abdominal bracing, keep your head on the floor and practice the breathing rhythm with the muscle contraction.
 ▮ Place the hands behind the head to support the neck.

Mindfulness   Abdominal bracing is initiated by contracting the deep inner core to create an internal tension that builds strength and stability of the core. Stay focused on maintaining the feeling of bracing the core from the inside as you move into more advanced exercises.

Leg Lift Tabletop

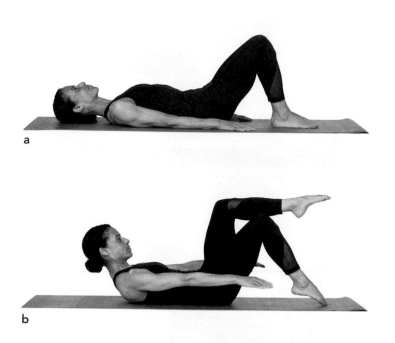

a

b

Starting Position Begin in the abdominal brace position (see figure a).

Action Curl up by bringing the ribs toward the hips to increase tension in the abdominal muscles. The shoulders are lifted off the floor and down and away from the ears. The hips are anchored to the floor as the ribs move toward the hips. Lift one leg at a time to bring both legs to a 90-degree angle in the hip and knee. Lower one leg to touch the toes to the floor (see figure b). Raise the leg back to the start position, and then repeat on the other leg. Brace the abdominal muscles as you lower the legs.

Alignment Be aware of the tendency for the abdominal muscles to pop out and the low back to hyperextend as you lift and lower the legs.

Breath Inhale to prepare. Exhale to contract the abdominal muscles and slide the ribs toward the hips. Inhale to lower the leg and exhale to lift. Repeat 6 to 12 times per side.

Progressions and Modifications
- To make this exercise easier, begin the leg lifts with the feet on the floor.
- To increase the challenge, lower both legs at one time.
- Vary the tempo by alternating the leg lifts, for greater challenge.

Mindfulness Brace the core without pushing the low back down. Become aware of just how much the abdominal muscles can work without compromising the low back.

Bend and Stretch

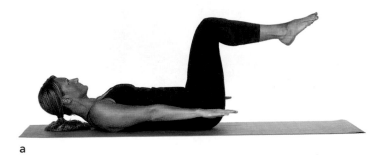

a

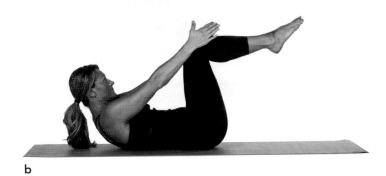

b

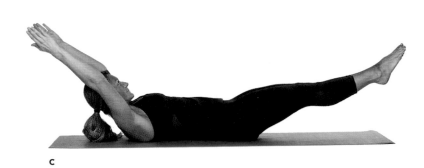

c

Starting Position   Begin in the abdominal brace position. Lift the legs to a 90-degree angle at the hip and knee and curl up, bringing the front of the ribs toward the hips (see figure *a*).

Action   Curl the upper body up, moving the front of the ribs toward the hips while keeping the hips anchored to the floor. Reach the arms to the knees with the palms turned in toward each other (see figure *b*). Reach the arms overhead as the legs extend out at a diagonal (see figure *c*). Circle the arms around to curl in to the start position.

Alignment   Maintain the abdominal brace position throughout the exercise by keeping the head lifted and the abdominal muscles pulled in and down.

Breath   Inhale to reach the arms and legs out. Exhale to contract the muscles of the core and bring the arms and legs to tabletop. Repeat 5 to 10 times.

Progressions and Modifications

- To make this exercise easier, perform the arm or leg action independently.
- To increase the challenge, lower the legs farther on the leg extension.
- Lower the head to the floor if there is discomfort in the neck.
- For variety, change the tempo by slowing the movement and taking slower and deeper breaths.

Mindfulness   Maintain the shape of your torso throughout the movement.

Single-Leg Stretch

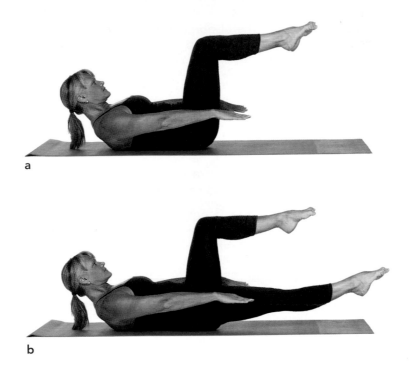

a

b

Starting Position   Begin in the abdominal brace position. Lift the legs to a 90-degree angle at the hip and knee and curl up, bringing the front of the ribs toward the hips. The hips are anchored to the floor as the ribs move toward the hips (see figure a).

Action   Curl up and reach the arms straight alongside the body and tuck the chin slightly. Extend one leg out straight (see figure b). Switch and stretch the opposite leg out straight.

Alignment   Maintain the abdominal brace position throughout the exercise. Avoid rocking the hips side to side.

Breath   Inhale to brace the core. Exhale to extend one leg out. Inhale to switch. Repeat 8 to 12 times per side.

Progressions and Modifications

- To make this exercise easier, keep the knee bent and touch the toe to the floor.
- To increase the challenge, place the hands behind the head.
- For variety, change the tempo by moving slower or quicker through the leg switches.

Mindfulness   Focus on the changes that occur in the muscles of the core that keep the movement graceful.

Crisscross

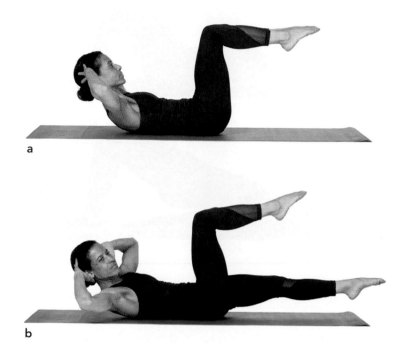

a

b

Starting Position   Begin in the abdominal brace position with the hands behind the head and the chin slightly tucked. Lift the legs to a 90-degree angle at the hip and knee and curl up, bringing the ribs toward the hips. The hips are anchored to the floor as the front of the ribs move toward the hips (see figure a).

Action   The shoulders lift slightly off the floor and press down and away from the ears as you curl up. Extend one leg out straight; at the same time, rotate the upper body toward the bent knee by moving the front ribcage to the opposite hip (see figure b). Switch to the opposite side.

Alignment   Maintain the abdominal brace position throughout the exercise. Avoid rocking the hips side to side.

Breath   Inhale to brace the core. Exhale to extend one leg out and rotate. Inhale to the center. Exhale to switch. Repeat 8 to 12 times per side.

Progressions and Modifications

- To make this exercise easier, keep the knee bent and touch the toe to the floor.
- For variety, change the tempo by moving slower or quicker through the leg switches.

Mindfulness   This exercise focuses on core connection rather than rotation. Imagine a crisscrossing of core muscle fiber like elastic strings reaching from the bottoms of the ribs to the opposite hip.

FOUNDATIONAL EXERCISE

Shoulder Bridge Position

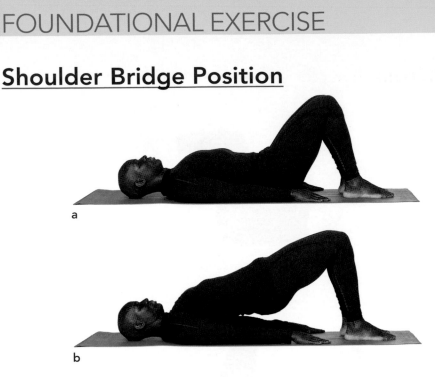

a

b

Starting Position   Lie on your back. The spine and pelvis are in a neutral alignment, the knees are bent, the feet are in line with the sitting bones, and the shins are in a vertical line. Place the arms on the floor at the side of the body (see figure *a*).

Action   Lengthen the back of the neck and bring the shoulder blades toward the center of the back. Press down into the feet to lift the hips and come onto the shoulder blades while maintaining a neutral spinal alignment (see figure *b*). Exert equal effort in the hamstrings, gluteals, and spinal muscles.

Alignment   Maintain neutral alignment of the spine from the shoulder blades to the knees as you lift and lower the hips.

Breath   Inhale to prepare. Exhale to lift to the shoulder bridge. Inhale and hold. Exhale to lower. Repeat 8 to 12 times.

Technique Tips

▮ Slide the bottom of the rib cage toward the hips to maintain a neutral back position.
▮ Slightly tuck the chin.
▮ Press into the inside edge of the feet to keep the knees aligned with the feet and hips.

Progressions and Modifications

▮ To increase intensity, reach the arms up toward the ceiling.
▮ Move the feet and legs together and squeeze the legs in as you lift up for more inner thigh work.
▮ For variety, hold the shoulder bridge in the lifted position for several breaths.

Mindfulness   Shoulder bridging is an excellent exercise for strengthening the muscles of the back of the body, particularly the gluteals and hamstrings. When performing this exercise, focus on the gluteal muscles initiating the movement. Be sure to keep them active throughout the exercise.

Shoulder Bridge With Leg Lift

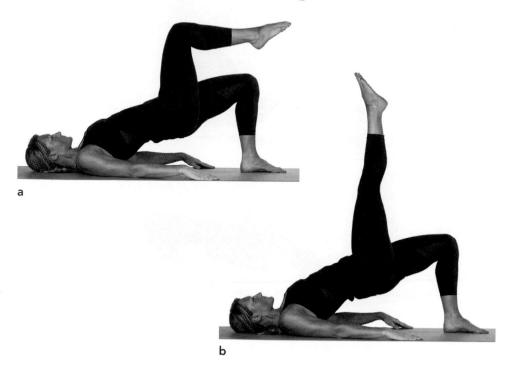

a

b

Starting Position   Begin in a shoulder bridge position. The spine and pelvis are in a neutral alignment, the knees are bent, the feet are in line with the sitting bones, and the shins are in a vertical line. Place the arms on the floor at the side of the body.

Action   Lengthen the back of the neck and bring the shoulder blades toward the center of the back. Lift one leg in a bent-knee position (see figure a). Press down into the supporting foot to lift the hips, coming onto the shoulder blades while maintaining a neutral spinal alignment. Exert equal effort in the hamstrings, gluteals, and spinal muscles. Lower the hips down keeping the leg lifted.

Alignment   Maintain neutral alignment of the spine from the shoulder blades to the knees as you lift and lower the hips. Avoid tilting the hips to one side.

Breath   Inhale to prepare. With one leg lifted, exhale to lift into the shoulder bridge. Inhale and hold. Exhale to lower. Repeat on one leg for 8 to 12 times per side.

Progressions and Modifications

- To increase the intensity, keep the lifted leg straight (see figure b).
- To increase the core challenge, in the shoulder bridge position, lift the leg with either a bent or straight knee, hold the shoulder bridge, and then lower and lift the leg three to five times before lowering out of the shoulder bridge.

Mindfulness   Place your hands on your hips to bring awareness to the shifting of the hips when one leg is lifted. Focus on keeping the hips level throughout the entire movement.

Shoulder Bridge in External Rotation

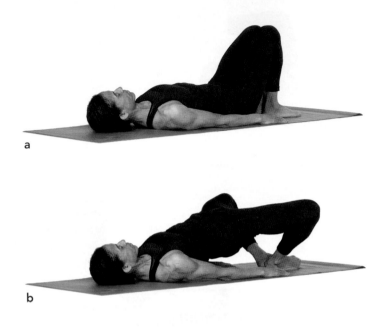

a

b

Starting Position   Begin in a shoulder bridge position. The spine and pelvis are in a neutral alignment, the knees are bent and the feet together, and the shins are in a vertical line. Place the arms on the floor at the side of the body (see figure a).

Action   Open the knees out to the side so that the outer edges of the feet are in contact with the floor. Keep tension in the legs and press down into the feet to lift the hips into a shoulder bridge (see figure b).

Alignment   Maintain neutral alignment of the spine. Exert equal effort in the hamstrings, gluteals, and spinal muscles.

Breath   Inhale to open the knee to the side. Exhale to lift the hips to the shoulder bridge. Inhale and hold. Exhale to lower. Repeat 8 to 12 times.

Progressions and Modifications
- To add more inner-thigh work, squeeze the inner thighs together as you lift and open as you lower.
- For variety, change the tempo and add a hold at the top.

Mindfulness   Slide the tailbone gently down toward the heels to create a sense of space in the low back. Keep the work equal in all of the muscles running up the back of the body.

7

Calming and Restorative Exercises

The exercises in this chapter calm and restore the body after your workout. This is an important part of your total workout and should not be left out. In fact, during cooling and recovery your body restores the physiological systems by bringing your nervous system, heart, lungs, muscles, and hormones back to their natural rhythm. This mirrors the thermostat in your home. The body has an ideal temperature setting that it maintains for normal function. During exercise the temperature in your internal thermostat rises. As you cool down the body comes back to its ideal temperature and setting. During recovery, your body has the time to restore, recharge, and rebuild and realize the physiological gains from the workout.

To begin the calming and restorative exercises, return to the intention you set at the beginning of the workout. Perhaps your intention was to complete one more repetition of each exercise. Another intention might be an increased focus on breath awareness. Return now to the intention and, without judgment, reflect on how your workout went.

To provide a more complete recovery, the exercises in this chapter are grouped according to movement intention. Select exercises from a variety of intention groups in order to achieve complete body recovery.

Stress and Weight Gain

If one of your goals for participating in a fusion workout is weight management, it is important to understand how mental anxiety and physical stress affect weight gain. When the body experiences eustress (positive stress) as in exercise, or distress (negative stress) as in worry, the body releases powerful hormones to combat it. These hormones give you greater energy and strength when you are involved in a physical workout. During the recovery phase of the workout, your body naturally lowers this hormonal level. Without recovery of perceived stress, these hormones remain in the bloodstream and begin to wreak havoc on the body. Two of the negative side effects are an increased release of insulin into the blood stream and increased fat storage (often in the midsection of the body). The body, in its brilliance, will store fat in the place it can most easily access it the next time you need it. This is why you need to spend the time practicing calming exercises in combination with the more physically challenging exercises. Many dietitians and nutritionists promote calming exercises as well as deep breathing for weight management.

Forward Bends

Forward bends are calming in general. The action of the torso moving forward and the closing of the front of the chest decreases the heart rate and slows the breathing rate. Notice this natural response in your body as you move in and out of forward bends.

Seated Forward Bend

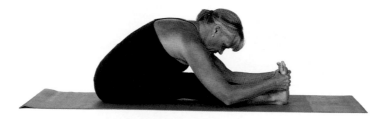

Starting Position   Begin in a seated position with the legs together straight out in front of the hips, and place the hands on the floor beside the hips. Sit on the center of the sitting bones and lift up through the spine to the top of the head.

Action   Hinge forward from the hips while maintaining a tall posture, taking the chest forward as the torso extends over the legs. Keep the shoulders relaxed. Lengthen the neck and keep the shoulders slightly back to open the front of the chest. Use the hands to help you to hinge forward by pressing them into the floor beside the hips. When you cannot hinge any farther, allow the spine to flex over the legs and the arms to reach toward the feet (see figure). If you can comfortably reach your feet, place the hands on the outsides of the feet. Relax into this position.

Alignment   Hinge forward from the hip and keep the spine in a long and length-ened position. Avoid excessive rounding of the upper back and lifting of the shoulders.

Breath   Inhale to sit tall. Exhale to move into the forward bend. Breathe naturally to relax. Focus on the exhalation to let go of unwanted tension. Hold for 5 to 10 deep breaths.

Progressions and Modifications
- Bend the knees slightly to help relax the hamstrings.
- Sit on a rolled mat or yoga block to elevate the hips and make it easier to bend forward.
- Place a yoga belt around the feet to help move deeper into the stretch.

Mindfulness   Bring awareness to the anatomical line along the back of the body. Begin on the bottom of the foot, travel up the back of the leg, and move over the hip and up the spine to your head. In a forward bend, you are lengthening this entire back line of the body.

Wide-Legged Forward Bend

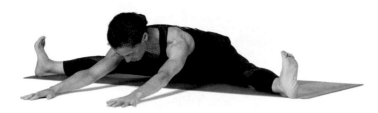

Starting Position Begin in a seated position with your legs straight out and in a V-shape. Your kneecaps point up, the ankles are flexed, and the toes point to the ceiling. Sit on the center of the sitting bones and lift through the spine through the top of the head. Place your hands on the floor in front of the torso.

Action Hinge forward while maintaining a tall posture, moving the torso forward and then toward the floor between the legs. Keep the shoulders relaxed and down and away from the ears. Maintain an open chest position. Use your hands to support yourself as you move the torso toward the floor. When you cannot hinge any farther, allow the spine to gently flex (see figure). Relax into this position.

Alignment As you hinge forward, keep the legs in the start position, with the knees pointed up toward the ceiling. Keep the shoulder relaxed down and the upper back long and extended.

Breath Inhale to sit tall. Exhale to move forward into the bend. Breathe naturally to relax. Focus on the exhalation to let go of unwanted tension. Hold for 5 to 10 deep breaths.

Progressions and Modifications

- Bend the knees slightly to help relax the hamstrings.
- Sit on a rolled mat or yoga block to elevate the hips to make it easier to bend forward.
- Place your hands behind your hips and press them into the floor to assist in hinging forward.

Mindfulness Focus your attention on the movement of the hips. The legs should stay still as you hinge forward, allowing the hips to rotate over the femur bones. Experience the sensation of lifting the sitting bones to move the torso forward.

Cross-Legged Seated Forward Bend

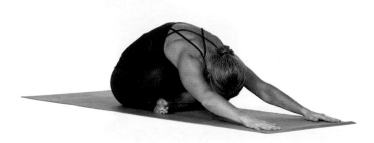

Starting Position   Begin in a seated position with your ankles crossed and hips open. Sit on the center of the sitting bones and lift through the spine to the top of the head.

Action   In the seated position, raise the arms above your head and hinge forward from the torso, bringing your hands to the floor. Gently curve the spine to complete the stretch (see figure). Relax into this position. Repeat with the opposite foot crossed in front.

Alignment   Use your hands to support your body as you hinge forward without putting tension on the neck and upper back.

Breath   Inhale to sit tall. Exhale to move into the forward bend. Inhale to expand the back of the rib cage, and exhale to relax. Hold for 5 to 10 deep breaths per side.

Progressions and Modifications

- Sit on a rolled mat or yoga block to elevate the hips to make it easier to open the hips and bend forward.
- In the forward bend position, with the hands on the floor reach one arm across to the opposite side to create a greater release of tension through the side and back of the torso. Repeat to the other side.

Mindfulness   You will feel the sensations of this stretch in many areas of your body. Observe where you hold tension and direct your breath into these places.

Puppy Pose

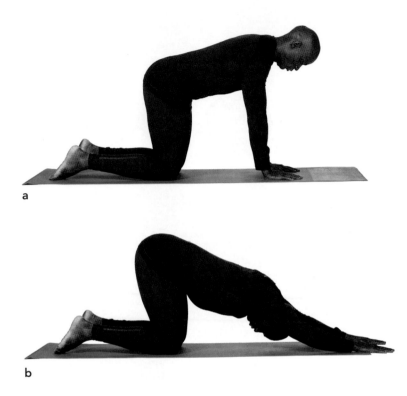

a

b

Starting Position Assume a kneeling position with your knees under the hips and the thighs in a vertical line (see figure a).

Action With the arms straight and shoulder-width apart, reach forward and lower the chest toward the floor while keeping the hips lifted (see figure b). The thighs are in a vertical line as the arms move forward and the chest lowers to the floor. Relax into this position.

Alignment Keep the deep abdominal muscles engaged to support the back and to prevent hyperextension of the spine.

Breath Inhale to initiate the movement. Exhale to lower the chest toward the floor. Hold for 5 to 10 deep breaths.

Progressions and Modifications

- Place a rolled mat under the knees for comfort.
- Bend the elbows and bring the forearms to the floor to decrease tension in the shoulders and back.

Mindfulness Focus on a deep and slow breathing rhythm to lower your heart rate and calm the body.

Twists

Twists penetrate deep into the core, offering benefits to the muscles of the torso and organs and creating suppleness and freedom in your spine. Practicing twists encourages deep and full breaths while detoxifying the body by removing the byproducts produced during exercise.

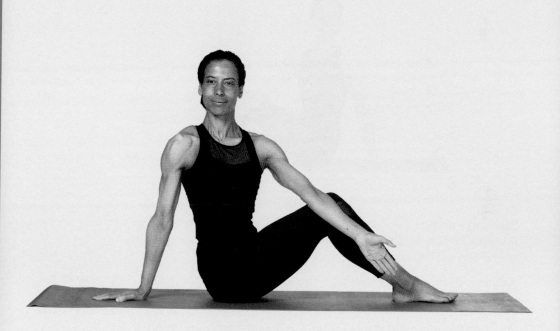

Seated Twist

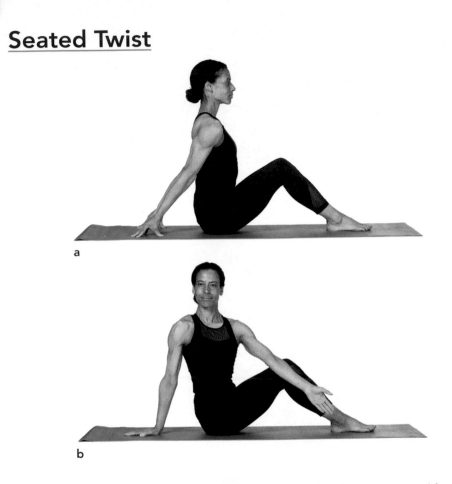

a

b

Starting Position   Assume a seated position with your knees bent and feet on the floor (see figure a). Sit on the center of the sitting bones and lift through the spine to the top of the head.

Action   Bring one arm overhead to create length on this side of the torso as the other hand presses into the floor to lift the spine. Keep the length of the spine as you rotate to the opposite side, maintaining a tall seated position and the rib cage close to the thigh. Bring the forearm across to the outer thigh and look over the back shoulder (see figure b). To assist with the twist, press gently into the thigh with the arm that reaches across the leg. Unwind slowly and repeat on the other side.

Alignment   Keep the spine long in a tall posture as you twist to the side. Keep the thighs on the centerline as you press the arm against the leg.

Breath   Inhale to sit tall. Exhale to rotate to one side. Breathe naturally. Hold for 5 to 10 deep breaths per side.

Progressions and Modifications

- Sit on a rolled mat or yoga block to elevate the hips for comfort.
- Lean the legs to one side to vary the seated twist.

Mindfulness   Breathe naturally. If your breath becomes labored, you have twisted too far.

Cross-Legged Seated Twist

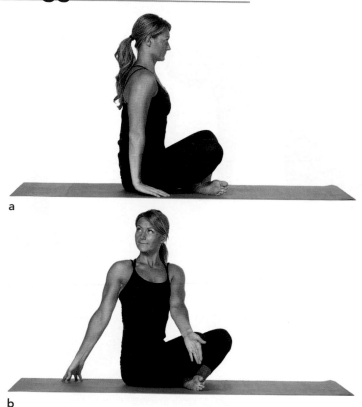

a

b

Starting Position   Begin in a cross-legged seated position. The knees are bent and one leg is folded under the opposite leg (see figure a). Sit on the center of the sitting bones and lift through the spine to the top of the head.

Action   Bring one arm overhead to create length on this side of the torso as the other hand presses into the floor to lift the spine. Keep the length in the spine as you rotate to the opposite side, maintaining a tall seated position and the rib cage close to the thigh. Bring your forearm across the outer thigh and look to the side (see figure b). Press gently into the thigh with the arm that reaches across the leg to assist with the twist. Unwind slowly and repeat on the other side.

Alignment   Keep the spine long in a tall posture as you twist to the side. Avoid letting the thigh fall inward as you press the arm into the thigh.

Breath   Inhale to sit tall. Exhale to rotate to one side. Breathe naturally. Hold for 5 to 10 deep breaths per side.

Progressions and Modifications

- Sit on a rolled mat or yoga block to elevate the hips for comfort.
- Straighten one leg in front and cross the other over in a bent-knee position if you feel discomfort in the knees.

Mindfulness   The twist should come from the ribs, upper back and neck while keeping equal weight on the sitting bones.

Kneeling Twist

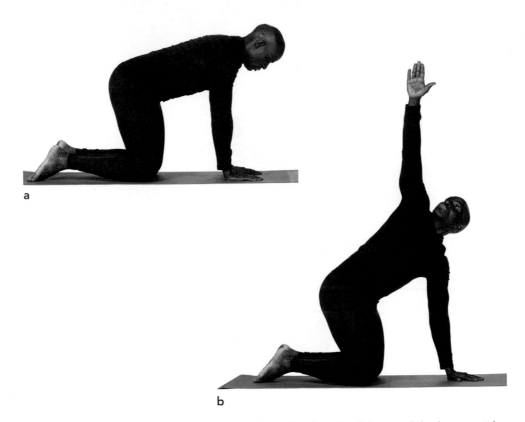

a

b

Starting Position   Kneel with your hands under the shoulders and the knees wider than the hips (see figure a).

Action   Place one hand on the floor in the midline of the body. Keeping the supporting arm straight, reach the opposite arm upward as the torso rotates to one side (see figure b). The eyes can look to the side or look up to the top hand.

Alignment   Keep the thighs in a vertical position and the supporting arm straight as you open the chest to one side in the rotation.

Breath   Inhale to set the position. Exhale to reach and rotate to one side. Breathe naturally. Hold for three to five breaths per side.

Progressions and Modifications
- Kneel on a folded towel or rolled mat for comfort.
- To decrease the intensity, wrap the arm around the back with the palm of the hand facing up rather than reaching the arm upward.

Mindfulness   This twist opens the front of the chest. Take time to notice how breath moves into the body more easily.

Revolving Low Lunge

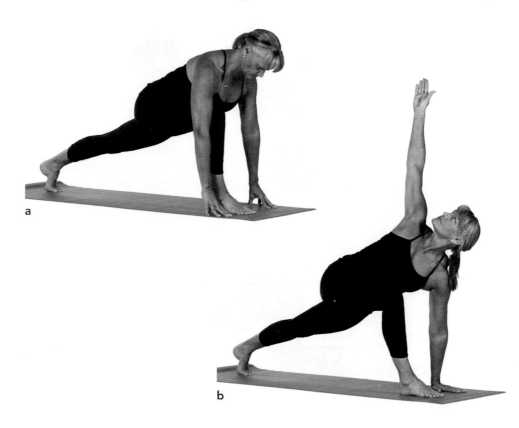

a

b

Starting Position   Assume a lunge position. The front leg creates a vertical line from the knee to the ankle and the back leg is extended straight back (see figure a).

Action   Place the opposite hand next to the front foot directly under the shoulder. Begin the rotation from the back hip and gently rotate through the spine to the top of the head. The rotation comes from the hips and moves into the upper body. At the same time, reach the free arm upward (see figure b). The head can turn to the side or look up to the top hand.

Alignment   Keep the knee of the forward leg aligned over the center of the foot and maintain length through the spine as you rotate.

Breath   Inhale to create length in the spine. Exhale to rotate to one side. Breathe naturally. Hold for 5 to 10 deep breaths per side.

Progressions and Modifications

- To decrease the intensity to the stretch, lower the back knee to the floor.
- Place a rolled mat under the knee for comfort.
- For variety, wrap the lifted arm around the back with the palm facing up.

Mindfulness   Open the chest and sense the length through the spine.

Thread the Needle

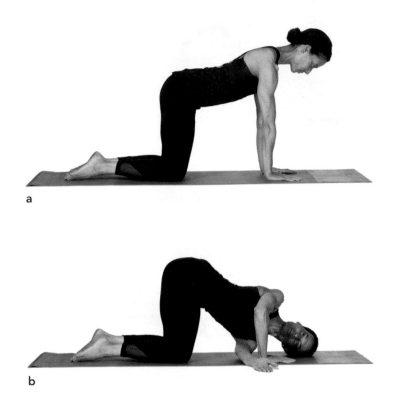

a

b

Starting Position   Assume a kneeling position. Your hands are under the shoulders and the knees are wider than the hips (see figure a).

Action   Reach one arm under the torso across to the opposite side with the palm of the hand turned up. Bring the outside of the shoulder to the floor and rest the side of the head on the floor (see figure b). The weight of the upper body is on the outer shoulder. The eyes can look to the side or look up to the top hand.

Alignment   Keep the thighs in a vertical position and the hips lifted. The rotation comes from the ribs and midback.

Breath   Inhale to lift the arm. Exhale to reach under and rotate to the side. Breathe naturally. Hold for 5 to 10 deep breaths per side.

Progressions and Modifications

- Kneel on a rolled mat for comfort.
- To create more rotation, keep the hand on the floor and press the fingers down rather than reaching the arm upward.
- Once the shoulder is on the floor, raise the opposite arm up.

Mindfulness   Focus on an even rhythm between the inhalation and exhalation.

Reclining Twist

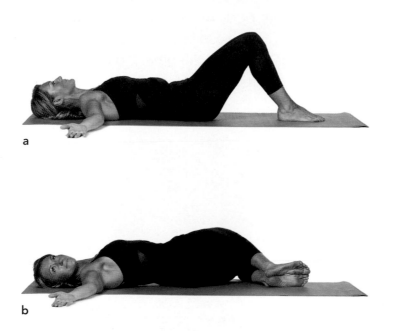

a

b

Starting Position   Lie on your back with the knees bent and feet on the floor. Open the arms out to the sides at shoulder height with the palms facing up (see figure a).

Action   With the legs together, rotate both legs to one side while keeping the shoulders on the floor (see figure b). Bring the legs back to center, and repeat in the opposite direction.

Alignment   Keep the shoulder blades on the floor as you rotate the legs to the side.

Breath   Inhale to prepare. Exhale to rotate to one side. Inhale to come back up. Exhale to the opposite side. Breathe naturally. Hold for three to five breaths per side.

Progressions and Modifications

- To increase the stretch, rotate to the side and straighten the top leg to reach the foot in front of the hip while in rotation.
- Lift both feet off the floor to rotate to one side. Keep them off the floor as you lift to go to the opposite side.

Mindfulness   This rotational stretch is about feeling good, so enjoy it.

Hip Releases

Tight hips affect almost all movements by limiting the range of motion and comfort during lower-body movements. Tight hips increase the strain on the low back, causing discomfort. Opening the hips and releasing tension brings energy to this area and can release stored-up negative feelings and emotions.

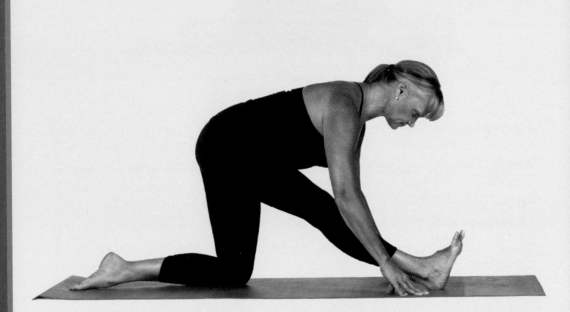

Low Lunge

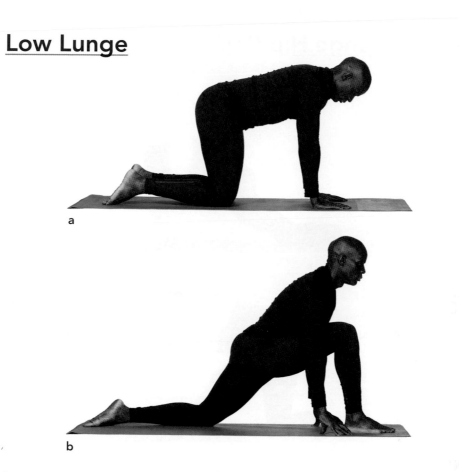

a

b

Starting Position Kneel with your hands under the shoulders and the knees under the hips (see figure a).

Action Step one foot forward to a lunge, placing the foot under the knee to create a vertical line along the shin. The knee of the front leg aligns directly over the ankle. The back leg can be straight or the knee can remain on the floor (see figure b).

Alignment Keep the spine long and the head in line with the spine. When the back knee is lifted off the floor, contract the muscles on the front of the thigh to support the knee joint.

Breath Inhale to set the position. Exhale to lower into the low lunge. Breathe naturally. Hold for three to five breaths per side.

Progressions and Modifications

- Kneel with the back knee on a rolled mat for comfort.
- Bring the hands on the inside of the front foot for a deeper stretch.
- Lower the back knee to the floor to decrease the effort and stretch.
- Step the front foot to the outside of the shoulder to open the inner thigh as well as stretch the hip flexors.
- Bring the arms overhead to create a stretch through the entire front of the body.

Mindfulness This is a deep stretch for the front of the hip and leg. Move slowly and gradually into this stretch to allow more time to relax.

Dynamic Lunge Hip Rock

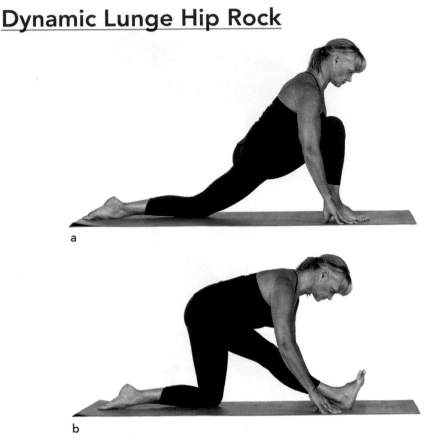

a

b

Starting Position Assume a lunge position with the knee of the front leg aligned directly over the ankle and the back knee on the floor (see figure a). The hands are on either side of the front foot.

Action Slowly move the hips back to straighten the front knee as you hinge the torso over the leg into a hamstring stretch (see figure b). Hold for a breath then move forward to the lunge. Hold the lunge for a breath and repeat, moving back to the hamstring stretch.

Alignment Keep the spine long as you rock the hips back into the hamstring stretch. The hips stay lifted, with the thigh in a vertical line for the hamstring stretch.

Breath Inhale into the lunge. Exhale to rock back into the hamstring stretch. Rock forward and back three to five times per side.

Progressions and Modifications

- Place a rolled mat under the back knee for comfort.
- Bring the arms up overhead in the lunge to create a stretch through the entire front of the body.
- Step the front foot to the outside of the shoulder to open the inner thigh and to stretch the hip flexors.

Mindfulness Create a rhythm between the breath and movement, using the full inhalation and exhalation to help move you from one position to the next.

Pigeon

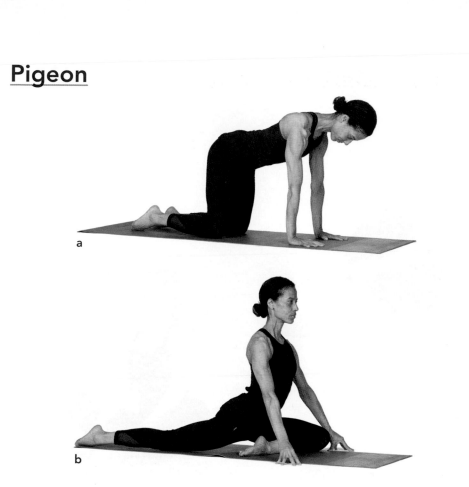

a

b

Starting Position Kneel with your hands under the shoulders and the knees under the hips (see figure *a*).

Action Bring one knee forward toward the chest, place the foot in front of the opposite hip crease, and rotate the hip out so that the leg is on the floor with the hip in this open position. Straighten the other leg back and lower the hips toward the floor. Support yourself with your hands on either side of your front knee (see figure *b*).

Alignment The back of the pelvis stays level. Avoid rolling to the bent-knee side; this puts undue strain on the knee.

Breath Inhale to bring the knee forward. Exhale to lower into pigeon pose. Breathe naturally. Hold for three to five breaths per side.

Progressions and Modifications

- For support in the pigeon pose, bring the forearms to the floor.
- If the hips are tilting to the side, place a block under the hip on the side of the bent knee.
- If it causes discomfort or pain in the knee, avoid doing this exercise.

Mindfulness Feel the stretch deep in the hips. Practice self-awareness and be honest with yourself. If this exercise causes more discomfort than potential gain, don't do the exercise. Most importantly, be okay with your decision. This is being mindful.

Seated Butterfly

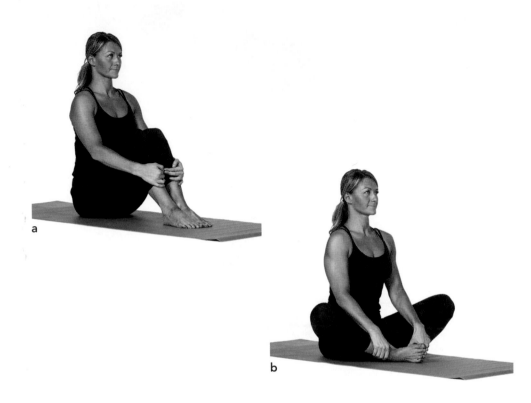

a

b

Starting Position   Begin in a seated position with your knees bent and feet on the floor. Sit on the center of the sitting bones and lift through the spine to the top of the head (see figure a).

Action   Remaining in a tall seated position, open the hips outward, move the knees to an open position, and place the hands on the ankles. Place the soles of the feet together (see figure b).

Alignment   The soles of both feet line up with each other. Stay centered on the sitting bones as the legs open out.

Breath   Inhale to sit tall. Exhale to open the legs. Breathe naturally. Hold for three to five breaths.

Progressions and Modifications

- Lean forward and press gently into the thighs with the arms to create a deeper stretch.
- Sit on a rolled mat or yoga block to elevate the hips for comfort.

Mindfulness   You may feel this exercise in the hips or back. Observe where you hold the most tension. Consciously relax into the stretch.

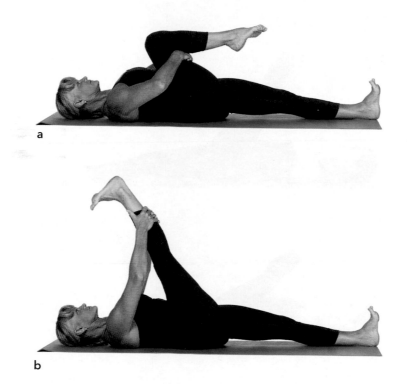

Reclining Hamstring Stretch

a

b

Starting Position   Lie on your back with one knee hugged into the chest and the other leg extended straight out on the floor. The ankle is flexed and the toes point up (see figure *a*).

Action   Hold onto the back of the bent leg and extend the leg upward to the extent of your flexibility without bending the opposite leg (see figure *b*). The heel of the lifted leg presses up.

Alignment   Ideally, both legs straighten; however, if your hamstrings are tight, bend the knee of the leg on the floor. The shoulders and shoulder blades stay on the floor. Avoid putting tension on the neck and shoulders.

Breath   Inhale to hug the knee to your chest. Exhale to extend the leg into the stretch. Breathe naturally. Hold for 5 to 10 deep breaths per side.

Progressions and Modifications

- Use a yoga belt around the foot of the extended leg to make the stretch more comfortable.
- For variety, bend and straighten the leg in a dynamic controlled rhythm.

Mindfulness   It is common to tense the neck and shoulders during this stretch. Be aware of relaxing this area. Place a soft smile on your face.

Reclining Adductor Stretch

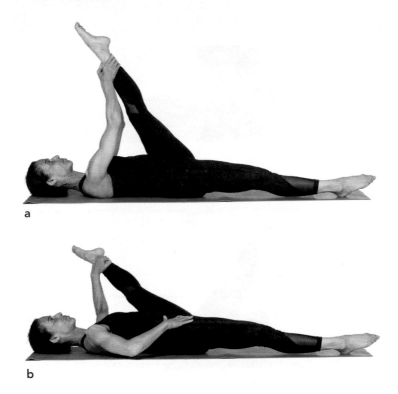

a

b

Starting Position   Lie on your back with one leg straight up and the other extended straight out on the floor. The ankle is flexed and the toes point up (see figure a).

Action   Hold onto the inside of the lifted leg; keep the leg straight and bring it out to the side (see figure b).

Alignment   Ideally, both legs are straight; however, if your hamstrings are tight, bend the knee of the leg you are stretching while keeping the other leg straight on the floor. The shoulders and the back of the hips stay on the floor. Avoid tension in the neck and shoulders.

Breath   Inhale to set the starting body position. Exhale to move the leg to the side. Breathe naturally. Hold for 5 to 10 deep breaths per side.

Progressions and Modifications

■ Use a yoga belt around the foot of the extended leg to make the stretch more comfortable.
■ For variety, move the leg out and in at a controlled rhythm.

Mindfulness   Bring your attention to the parts of the body that are in contact with the floor on the side of the body that is not being stretch. Keep the heel, calf, hip, shoulder blade, and head in contact with the floor.

Reclining Abductor Stretch

a

b

Starting Position Lie on your back with one leg straight up and the other extended straight out on the floor (see figure a). The ankles are flexed.

Action Keep the leg straight, and bring the leg across the body without lifting the hip off the floor. The leg crosses the midline of the body (see figure b).

Alignment Ideally, both legs are straight; however, if your hamstrings are tight, bend the knee of the leg you are stretching while keeping the other leg straight on the floor. The shoulders and shoulder blades stay on the floor. Avoid tension in the neck and shoulders.

Breath Inhale to set the starting body position. Exhale to bring the leg to the side. Breathe naturally. Hold for 5 to 10 deep breaths per side.

Progressions and Modifications

- To decrease the intensity of the stretch, bend the knee to cross the leg over to the side.
- For a deeper hip release, move the leg back and forth across the body in a controlled rhythm.

Mindfulness This stretch gets deep inside of the hip joint; take your time to sense where you feel the tension and breathe into the tightness.

Reclining Figure-4

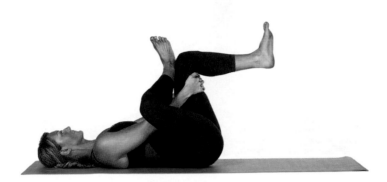

Starting Position   Lie on your back with your knees bent and feet on the floor.

Action   Place one foot across the thigh of the other leg. Flex the foot at the ankle and turn the hip out. Lift the opposite leg toward the chest (see figure).

Alignment   Keep the hips on the floor and avoid tension in the neck and shoulders.

Breath   Inhale to set the starting body position. Exhale to move into the stretch. Breathe naturally. Hold for 5 to 10 deep breaths per side.

Progressions and Modifications

- To decrease the intensity of the stretch, keep one foot on the floor.
- To focus on hip mobility, move the hips in a small circle in both directions.

Mindfulness   Take time to feel the hips and low back relax. Breathe.

Chest Releases

Most people are tight in the front of the shoulders and chest because of long hours of sitting while working on computers and driving and because of poor posture. You can do the chest-releasing exercises in this section anytime and anywhere. They are especially effective when you take a break from working or sitting for extended periods.

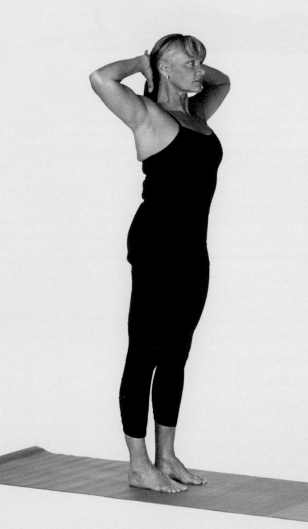

Supported Back Extension

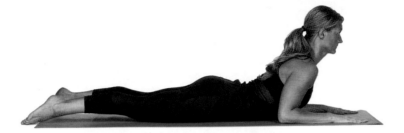

Starting Position   Lie facedown with the forearms on the floor beside the shoulders and the palms of the hands facing down. The legs are extended straight back, hip-distance apart, with the tops of the feet on the floor.

Action   Lift the abdominal wall toward the spine and contract the quadriceps to lift the kneecaps off the floor. Roll the shoulders back, and move the shoulder blades down the back as you lift the chest off the floor (see figure). Gently press upward with the arms. Lift the chest only as high as is comfortable for the low back. If you sense compression in the low back, lower the upper-body position.

Alignment   Keep the head in line with the natural curve of the spine. Avoid letting the head fall forward or hyperextend back.

Breath   Exhale to contract the quadriceps to lift the kneecaps and to set the core. Inhale to lift the chest. Breathe naturally. Hold for three to five deep breaths.

Progressions and Modifications
- Lift into the extension on an inhale and lower on the exhale in a slow controlled rhythm.
- For greater strengthening of the upper back as well as stretch for the chest, reach the fingers toward the feet as you lift into the back extension.

Mindfulness   Focus on opening the chest rather than extending the back. Imagine moving the sternum forward and lifting the chest creating a sense of space in the front of the body.

Seated Cow Face Pose

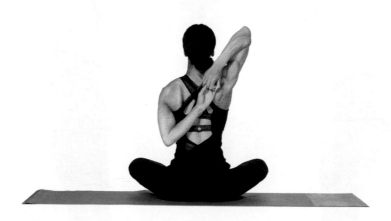

Starting Position   Assume a seated crossed-legged position centered on the sitting bones. Lift through the spine to the top of the head.

Action   Remaining in a tall seated position, reach one arm overhead. Bend the elbow and place the palm between the shoulder blades. Reach the opposite arm behind the back and bend the elbow to reach the hand up the back toward the other hand (see figure). Clasp the hands behind your back.

Alignment   Maintain a tall seated position as the arms move into the stretch. Tuck the chin slightly and press the head back into the arms to maintain good alignment of the head.

Breath   Inhale to bring the arms into place. Exhale to open the chest and move more deeply into the stretch. Breathe naturally. Hold for 5 to 10 deep breaths per side.

Progressions and Modifications

- To decrease the intensity of the stretch, reach one arm behind the head and use the opposite arm to hold onto the elbow to bring the arm into the stretch.
- Standing to do the exercise can make it easier to achieve the range of motion.
- For comfort, sit on a yoga block to give the hips more mobility to sit cross-legged.

Mindfulness   Relax through the neck and shoulder.

Dynamic Four-Point Stretch

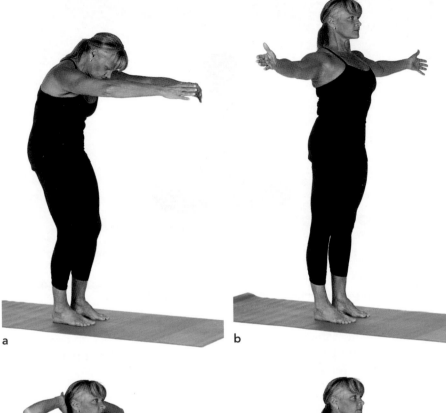

a

b

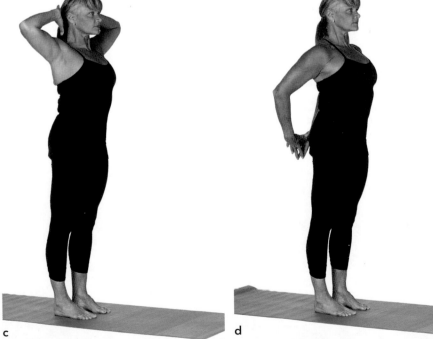

c

d

Starting Position   Stand tall. Reach the arms in front of the chest and, at the same time, round the upper back (see figure *a*).

Action   Move the arms straight out from the shoulders and slightly extend the upper back (see figure *b*). Bring the hands behind the head, lifting the elbows up and back (see figure *c*). Sweep the arms down and behind the hips to touch the fingers together (see figure *d*).

Alignment   Maintain a tall posture through the legs and hips. Allow the upper body to move freely with the movement of the arms.

Breath   Exhale to bring the arms forward. Inhale to reach the arms out. Exhale to bring the hands behind the head. Inhale to reach the arms behind the back. Repeat the sequence three to five times.

Progressions and Modifications

- Move the arms through a pain-free range of motion.
- To add a sense of calm, hold each arm position for a few breaths before moving to the next position.

Mindfulness   Move with grace and freedom.

Side Bends

Side bending releases tension through the lateral line of the body. This often forgotten movement is important for overall spinal health. These exercises aid in releasing tension in the back and keep the spine mobile.

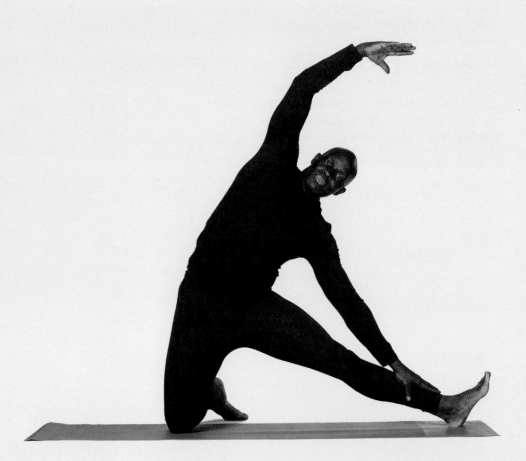

Seated Side Bend

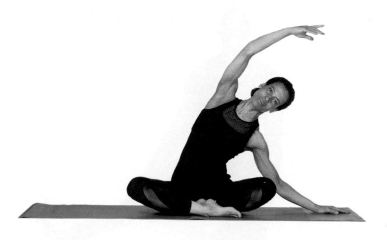

Starting Position   Assume a seated crossed-legged position centered on the sitting bones and lifted through the spine to the top of the head.

Action   Stay in a tall seated position and reach one arm overhead. Continue to reach the arm over into a side bend through the torso (see figure). Repeat on the other side as you reach the opposite arm over in a dynamic sweeping motion.

Alignment   Keep the hips equally weighted down. Avoid rounding forward.

Breath   Inhale to bring the arm overhead. Exhale to bend to the side. Inhale to return to the center. Exhale to bend to the other side. Repeat three to five times.

Progressions and Modifications

- Change the leg position if sitting crossed legged is uncomfortable.
- Sit on a yoga block for comfort.
- If seated causes tension in the low back, stand to perform the exercise.

Mindfulness   Imagine your upper body is moving between two panes of glass.

Kneeling Side Bend

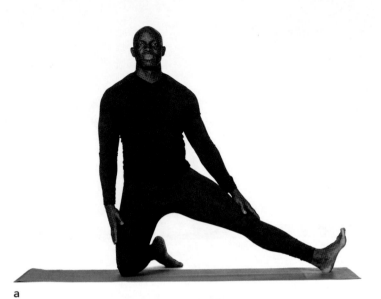

a

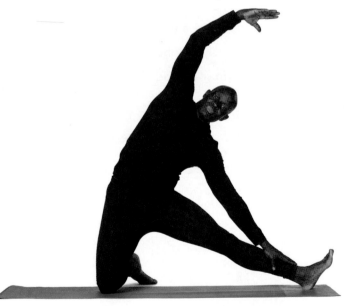

b

Starting Position   Begin by kneeling on both knees. Extend one leg out to the side. The knee and toe are pointed up. Bring the upper body into an upright position (see figure *a*).

Action   Maintaining a tall position, reach the opposite arm overhead and bend to the side toward the straight leg (see figure *b*). Reach the opposite arm over in a sweeping motion to reach in the opposite direction. Move from side to side in a dynamic and controlled manner. After completing repetitions on one side; repeat on the other side.

Alignment   Keep the hips level. Avoid rounding forward. The knee of the extended leg is pointed up throughout the movement.

Breath   Inhale to bring the arm overhead. Exhale to bend to the side. Inhale to return to the center. Exhale to bend to the other side. Repeat three to five times.

Progressions and Modifications
  ▌ Kneel on a rolled yoga mat for comfort on the knee.
  ▌ Keep both knees bent in the kneeling position if the stretch is uncomfortable in the hip.

Mindfulness   Link your breath and movement to create a gentle flow.

Soothing Exercises

Soothing exercises calm the body by lowering the heart rate, by lowering blood pressure, and by slowing your breathing. Practice these exercises any time you feel the need to restore your energy and calm your mind.

Child's Pose

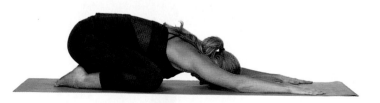

Starting Position Kneel with the knees about shoulder-width apart and the inside edges of the feet together.

Action Reach the arms forward, shoulder-width apart. Sit the hips back to the heels, bringing your ribs to the inside of the thigh. Keep the arms straight and lower the chest toward the floor (see figure).

Alignment The arms are extended with the elbows lifted off the floor and without tension in the shoulders. The spine is in a gentle and relaxed curve from the hips to the head.

Breath Inhale to initiate the movement. Exhale to lower into the stretch. Hold for 5 to 10 deep breaths.

Progressions and Modifications

- Place a rolled mat under the knees for comfort.
- Bring the arms to the side of the body with the palms of the hands facing up for a more relaxed position.
- Place a yoga block under the forehead to decrease tension in the back of the neck.

Mindfulness Focus on a deep, slow breathing rhythm to lower your heart rate and calm the body. Sense the movement of the rib cage gently expanding and contracting with each breath.

Calm Lake

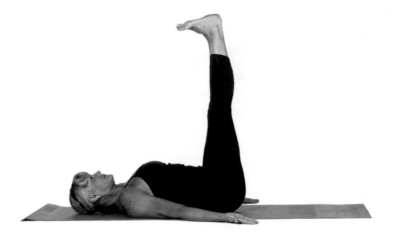

Starting Position   Lie on your back with both legs extended straight up. The arms are beside the body in a comfortable position and the palms turned up.

Action   Flex the ankles and gently pull the toes down toward the shins (see figure). Ideally, both legs are straight; however, if the hamstrings and low back are tight, bend the knees to release the tension.

Alignment   The shoulders and shoulder blades stay on the floor. The head and neck are in a neutral alignment and the tip of the nose points up.

Breath   Inhale to extend the legs up. Exhale to settle into the stretch. Breathe naturally. Hold for 5 to 10 deep breaths.

Progressions and Modifications

- Place the legs up a wall for greater relaxation.
- Wrap a yoga belt around the leg at midthigh and gently pull to decrease the work of the leg muscles and increase relaxation.
- Bend the knees toward the chest to decrease the effort.

Mindfulness   Close your eyes and take your focus into your inner world, to the sensations of your body and the thoughts in your mind. Imagine a calm lake and let the mind and body come to this place.

Reclining Knee-Hug Stretch

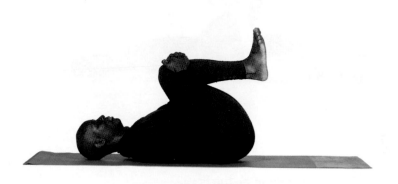

Starting Position Lie on your back and pull both knees toward the chest. The arms are beside the body in a comfortable position with the palms turned up.

Action Wrap the arms around the shins and gently pull the knees into the chest (see figure).

Alignment The shoulders and shoulder blades are on the floor and the neck is relaxed.

Breath Inhale to hug the knees into your chest. Exhale to relax. Breathe naturally. Hold for 5 to 10 deep breaths.

Progressions and Modifications
- Rock the knees in and out to massage the low back.
- Roll the hips side to side to release tension in the back.

Mindfulness Focus on the low back and let go of tension with each exhalation.

Reclining Single-Leg Hug Stretch

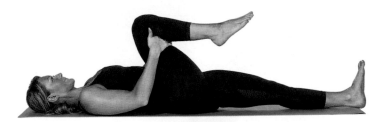

Starting Position   Lie on your back with one knee hugged into the chest and the other leg extended straight out on the floor.

Action   Wrap the arms around the back of the thigh and gently pull the knee in closer to the chest (see figure).

Alignment   Keep the back of the body from the head to the heel of the straight leg on the floor in a straight line.

Breath   Inhale to hug the knee into your chest. Exhale to relax. Breathe naturally. Hold for 5 to 10 deep breaths per side.

Progressions and Modifications
- To increase hip mobility, place the hand on the knee and circle the bent knee in one direction and then the other direction.
- Bend the straight leg and place the foot on the floor if you feel discomfort in your low back.

Mindfulness   Focus on the rhythm of your breath. Take in a slow relaxed inhalation and a long exhalation.

Reclining Butterfly

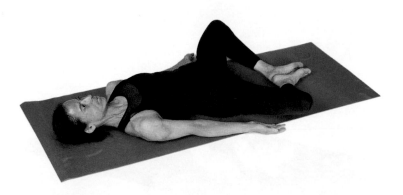

Starting Position   Lie on the back with the knees bent and feet on the floor. Reach the arms along the sides of the body with the palms facing up in a comfortable position.

Action   Open the hips by moving the knees out and placing the bottoms of the feet together (see figure).

Alignment   The back of the hips, shoulders, and shoulder blades are on the floor as the legs open out. The neck is relaxed.

Breath   Inhale to bend the knees. Exhale to open the knees and relax into the stretch. Breathe naturally. Hold for 5 to 10 deep breaths.

Progressions and Modifications

- Place a yoga block under both knees to support the legs and relax more deeply into this stretch.
- Pull the heels in closer to the hips for a greater hip stretch.

Mindfulness   Breathe slowly and deeply, allowing your energy to settle into a state of peacefulness.

Happy Baby

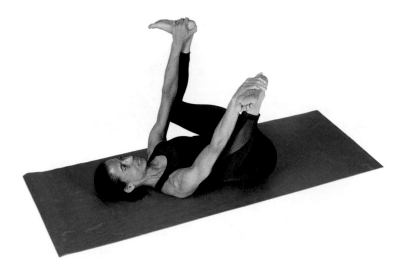

Starting Position Lie on your back, bend the knees toward the chest, and hold the insides of the feet with the hands.

Action Open the hips and bring the knees down toward the sides and shoulders (see figure).

Alignment The shoulders and shoulder blades are on the floor as the legs open out. The neck is relaxed.

Breath Inhale to bend the knees. Exhale to pull the legs into the stretch. Breathe naturally. Hold for 5 to 10 deep breaths.

Progressions and Modifications
- Rock side to side to release and relax the low back.
- For a deeper stretch on one side of the body, open one hip at a time by bringing one leg up while the other foot stays on the floor. Repeat on the other side.

Mindfulness Remember when you were a child without a care in the world; bring that memory to this release.

Resting Pose

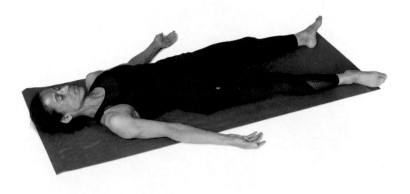

Starting Position   Lie on your back with the legs straight and the arms at the side of the body and the palms facing up.

Action   Let the muscles of the hips and low back relax, allowing the legs to naturally roll out (see figure). The back of the hips, shoulders, and shoulder blades are on the floor with the neck relaxed.

Alignment   The spine is in a neutral alignment from the head to the toes.

Breath   Inhale to open the chest. Exhale to relax. Breathe naturally. Hold for 10 to 20 deep breaths, or set a timer and stay in resting pose for 5 to 10 minutes.

Progressions and Modifications

- To decrease tension in the low back, bend the knees and lean the inner thighs against each other.
- Lie on your side with the knees comfortably bent if lying on your back causes discomfort.
- Place a rolled towel under the knees to decrease tension in the back.

Mindfulness   Let your mind and body completely relax. Allow yourself to surrender to gravity, letting go of all muscular effort. Allow the mind to rest as much as the body. As thoughts come to mind, allow them to float away without attachment. Clear the mind and find peace. Your list of things to do can wait until after this important resting pose.

Fusion Workout System

BY LEVEL

BY TIME

BY PURPOSE

BY ACTIVITY

Never be bored with your workout routine again. In the following chapters you will see the diversity of the fusion workout system. Choose from the 15 sample workouts to find your perfect workout for the day.

The fusion workout system is designed to meet your ever-changing needs and can easily be adjust based on your purpose and the amount of time you have to workout. In the following chapters are sample workouts based on fitness level, time, purpose for training, and preferred activity. Once you become comfortable with the workouts, you can tweak them by adding exercises, changing the number of repetitions or time, and choosing a different variation of the exercise from the fusion exercise library in chapters 4 through 7.

Use the workouts in this book or design your own unique workout simply by following the fusion workout system and template in appendix A and selecting exercises from each of the exercise categories in the fusion workout exercise chapters.

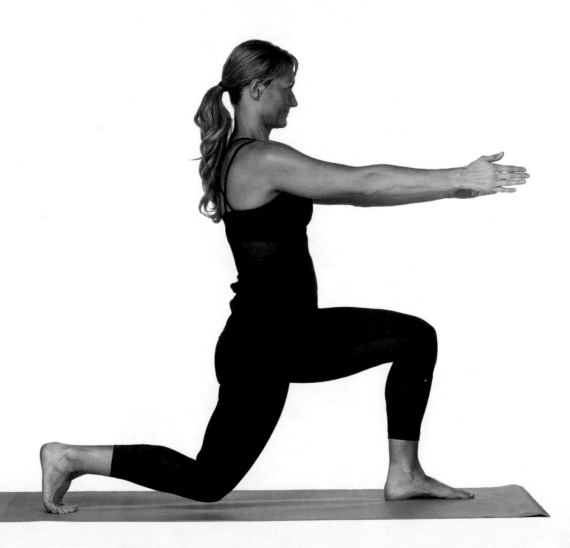

8

Fusion Workouts
∎ BY LEVEL

The fusion workouts in this chapter are based on intensity. The exercises, duration and number of repetitions change in each level to progressively become more challenging. Each level can progress gradually to the next level by increasing the number of repetitions you perform and the length of time you hold the exercise. Before each workout you may want to refresh your memory by referring to the previous chapters for technique suggestions as well as for progression and modifications. Many of the warm-up exercises in chapter 4 and the calming and restorative exercises in chapter 7 can be used for either warming up or calming down. In the workout charts that follow, you will see these exercises used in either step of the workout; refer to the page numbers for reference. The mindful exercises from chapter 3 appear in the sample workouts.

The begin fusion workout is an excellent place to start or a good workout to come back to if you have had an extended time away from exercise. When you begin exercising, do this workout three times per week and gradually work your way up to daily. When you feel this workout is no longer challenging, move to the next level. As you move to the more challenging workouts, you can still come back to this workout on days that you need less challenge or are tight on time.

Move through the exercises at your own pace. When you become fatigued, take a break before moving on. Progress to more challenging variations of the exercises when you feel ready to take on more work.

Intention: Take your time to master the exercises and gain confidence. Focus on good form, alignment, and exercise execution. Concentrate on the quality of the exercise rather than the quantity.

	Exercise	Page #	Time or reps	Exercise recommendations and variations
Warm-up (10 min.)	Seated 3D breathing	13	1 min.	Center your mind and body using 3D breathing.
	Puppy pose	126	Hold for 3-5 breaths.	
	Cat and cow stretch	30	Move from cat to cow at a controlled pace for 3-5 reps.	
	Low lunge	135	Hold the lunge on each side for 3-5 breaths.	Perform with hands off the floor.
Transition	**From kneeling, press back toward the feet and lift the knees, coming into a standing forward bend with the knees bent. Slowly roll up to standing.**			

	Exercise	Page #	Time or reps	Exercise recommendations and variations
Warm-up (contd.)	**Mountain pose with arms reaching**	42	Hold for 3-4 breaths.	
	Fusion sun salutation flow 1	45	3-4 reps	
Standing fusion exercises (15 min.)	**Squat**	50	8-12 reps	Move at a tempo of 2-4 counts to lower and stand up.
	Lunge	60	8-12 reps on each side	Move at a tempo of 2-4 counts to lower and stand up.
	Single-leg balance	72	Hold for 3-5 deep breaths on each side.	

> continued

	Exercise	Page #	Time or reps	Exercise recommendations and variations
	Warrior 2 (R)	66	Hold for 3-5 breaths.	
	Reverse warrior (R)	68	Hold for 3-5 breaths.	
	Warrior 2 (L)	66	Hold for 3-5 breaths.	
	Reverse warrior (L)	68	Hold for 3-5 breaths.	
Transition	**Perform a standing forward bend and step back to plank.**			
Floor fusion exercises (15 min.)	**Wide push-up**	89	6-12 reps	Support weight on knees or toes.
	Plank Position	37	Hold for 3-5 breaths.	Support weight on forearms.

Exercise		Page #	Time or reps	Exercise recommendations and variations
Side plank		90	Hold for 3-5 breaths on each side.	Support weight on forearm. Perform with bent knee or straight leg.
Two-point tabletop		92	Hold for 3-5 breaths on each side.	Alternate the arm and leg lift.
Back extension		94	3-5 reps	Place hands on the floor. Lift and lower at a controlled tempo.
Hip extension		98	3-5 reps	Lift and lower at a controlled tempo.
Half rollback		102	3-5 reps	Place hands behind the thighs for support.
V-sit		104	Hold for 3-5 breaths.	Feet are on the floor.
Abdominal brace position		112	3-5 reps	Lift and lower at a controlled tempo.
Leg lift tabletop		113	3-5 reps	Alternate each leg lift and lower at a controlled tempo.
Shoulder bridge position		118	Hold for 3-5 breaths.	Add more repetitions to increase the intensity.

> continued

	Exercise	Page #	Time or reps	Exercise recommendations and variations
Calming and restorative exercises (10 min.)	**Reclining knee-hug stretch**	155	Hold for 5 breaths.	
	Reclining twist	133	Hold for 5 breaths on each side.	
	Reclining hamstring stretch	139	Hold for 5 breaths on each side.	Perform on both legs.
	Reclining figure-4	142	Hold for 5 breaths on each side.	
	Calm lake	154	Hold for 5 breaths.	
	Resting pose	159	Hold for 1 to 5 min.	Take this time to congratulate yourself for doing the work. Give yourself permission to enjoy the rest.

The evolve fusion workout is an intermediate-level workout that will challenge strength, balance, and flexibility. This workout is perfect if you are ready to try more challenging variations of the exercises in the fusion workout method. When you begin this level of fusion workouts, add one per week while continuing the begin-level fusion workouts on the other days. As your fitness improves, replace the begin-level workouts with more evolve-level workouts per week. When this workout becomes easy for you, move to the challenge-level fusion workout.

Intention: Proper technique and good form determine whether an exercise is effective and safe. Focus on the foundation of each exercise. Ensure that your foundation is well set so that you can execute the rest of the movement with good alignment.

	Exercise	Page #	Time or reps	Exercise recommendations and variations
Warm-up (10 min.)	Child's pose	29	Hold for 5 breaths.	Practice 3D breathing with a focus on expanding the back of the rib cage.
	Cat and cow stretch	30	3-5 reps	Move from cat to cow at a controlled pace.
	Low lunge to kneeling hamstring stretch	34	3-5 reps on each side	Move from the lunge with the hands on the floor to the hamstring stretch at a controlled tempo.
	Plank position	37	Hold for 3-5 breaths.	Support weight on bent knee or on toes.
	Downward-facing dog	38	Hold for 3-5 breaths.	Substitute child's pose as an option.

> continued

	Exercise	Page #	Time or reps	Exercise recommendations and variations
Transition	Step the feet forward to the hands as you move into a standing forward bend.			
Warm-up (contd.)	**Mountain pose with arms reaching**	42	3-4 reps	
	Fusion sun salutation flow 2	46	3-4 reps	
Standing fusion exercises (15 min.)	**Squat**	50	8 to 12 reps	Move at a tempo of 2-4 counts to lower and stand up.
	Chair pose	54	Hold for 5 breaths.	
	Lunge (R)	60	5 to 8 reps	Move at a tempo of 2-4 counts to lower and stand up.

Exercise		Page #	Time or reps	Exercise recommendations and variations
Crescent lunge (R)		64	Hold for 3-5 breaths.	
Warrior 2 (R)		66	Hold for 3-5 breaths.	
Reverse warrior (R)		68	Hold for 3-5 breaths.	
Extended side angle (R)		70	Hold for 3-5 breaths.	
Lunge (L)		60	5 to 8 reps	Move at a tempo of 2-4 counts to lower and stand up.

> continued

Exercise	Page #	Time or reps	Exercise recommendations and variations
Crescent lunge (L)	64	Hold for 3-5 breaths.	
Warrior 2 (L)	66	Hold for 3-5 breaths.	
Reverse warrior (L)	68	Hold for 3-5 breaths.	
Extended side angle (L)	70	Hold for 3-5 breaths.	
Single-leg balance (R)	72	Hold for 3-5 breaths.	

Exercise	Page #	Time or reps	Exercise recommendations and variations
Side balance (R)	74	Hold for 3-5 breaths.	
Single-leg balance (L)	72	Hold for 3-5 breaths.	
Side balance (L)	74	Hold for 3-5 breaths.	
Transition	**Perform a standing forward bend and step back to plank.**		
Floor fusion exercises (20 min.)	**Plank position**	37	Hold for 3-5 breaths.	
	Plank with leg lift	83	5 reps on each side	Alternate the leg lifts from right to left. Link the movement with the breath.
	Narrow push-up	88	5-10 reps	Support weight on the knees or toes.

> continued

Exercise	Page #	Time or reps	Exercise recommendations and variations
Side plank	90	Hold for 5 breaths on each side.	Support weight on hand or forearm.
Two-point tabletop (R)	92	Hold for 3-5 breaths.	Alternate arm and leg lift.
Two-point tabletop (R)	92	Hold for 3-5 breaths.	Alternate arm and leg lift to the side.
Two-point tabletop (L)	92	Hold for 3-5 breaths.	Alternate arm and leg lift.
Two-point tabletop (L)	92	Hold for 3-5 breaths.	Alternate arm and leg lift to the side.
Back extension	94	3-5 reps	Hands are at the forehead. Lift and lower at a controlled tempo.
Hip extension	98	3-5 reps	Lift and lower at a controlled tempo.
Half rollback	102	3-5 reps	Perform an oblique half rollback by alternating sides.
V-sit	104	Hold for 3-5 breaths.	Keep feet on the floor.

	Exercise	Page #	Time or reps	Exercise recommendations and variations
	Reverse table	105	Hold for 3-5 breaths.	Perform with bent knees.
	Side leg lift	107	5-10 reps on each side	
	Abdominal brace position	112	3-5 reps	Hands are behind the head. Lift and lower at a controlled tempo.
	Single-leg stretch	116	5-10 reps on each side	Alternate legs.
	Shoulder bridge with leg lift	119	Hold for 3-5 breaths.	Perform with bent knee or straight leg.
Calming and restorative exercises (10 min.)	**Reclining single-leg hug stretch (R)**	156	Hold for 5 breaths.	
	Reclining twist (R)	133	Hold for 5 breaths.	Perform with single leg.
	Reclining hamstring stretch (R)	139	Hold for 5 breaths.	

> continued

Exercise	Page #	Time or reps	Exercise recommendations and variations
Reclining figure-4 (R)	142	Hold for 5 breaths.	
Reclining single-leg hug stretch (L)	156	Hold for 5 breaths.	
Reclining twist (L)	133	Hold for 5 breaths.	Perform with single leg.
Reclining hamstring stretch (L)	139	Hold for 5 breaths.	
Reclining figure-4 (L)	142	Hold for 5 breaths.	
Happy baby	158	Hold for 3-5 breaths.	
Calm lake	154	Hold for 5 breaths.	
Progressive relaxation		Flow through the entire body one time.	
Resting pose	159	Hold for 3-5 min.	Congratulate yourself for doing this workout. Be proud.

CHALLENGE LEVEL WORKOUT

The challenge fusion workout is the most intense of the fusion workout levels. Do this workout when you are ready to push yourself to the next level of fitness. Add one challenge fusion workout into your weekly fitness routine as you progress from the evolve-level fusion workouts. Gradually increase the number of times you do this workout up to four days per week. On the other days of the week, do easier fusion workouts. At first, start with the easier version of the exercise and progress to challenge yourself to perform the most advanced option. As your skill level increases, add more repetitions or hold the exercise for a longer time. Once the challenge fusion workout becomes familiar and you are ready for variety, you can add other fusion exercises from chapters 4 through 7 into this workout.

Intention: Use breath control to give you strength when you need it and to foster relaxation when you are holding on too tightly. The inhalations bring energy into the body, and the exhalations help release unwanted tension. Focus on strong, deep breaths.

	Exercise	Page #	Time or reps	Exercise recommendations and variations
Warm-up (10 min.)	**Child's pose**	29	Hold for 5 deep breaths.	Practice 3D breathing with a focus on expanding the back of the rib cage.
	Cat and cow stretch	30	5 reps	Move from cat to cow at a controlled pace.
	Spinal rotation with thread the needle	32	3 reps on each side	Move with the inhalation to rotate, and during the exhalation, move into thread the needle. Hold thread the needle for 2-3 breaths before rotating again.
	Plank position	37	Hold for 3-5 breaths.	Support weight on knees or toes.

> continued

Exercise	Page #	Time or reps	Exercise recommendations and variations
Downward-facing dog	38	Hold for 3-5 breaths.	
Low lunge to kneeling hamstring stretch	34	3-5 reps on each side	Move from the lunge with the hands on the floor to the hamstring stretch at a controlled tempo. Bring the arms overhead on the lunge.
Plank position	82	Hold for 3-5 breaths.	Support weight on knees or toes.
Downward-facing dog	38	Hold for 3-5 breaths.	
Transition	**Step the feet forward to the hands as you move into a standing forward bend.**		
Warm-up (contd.)	**Mountain pose with arms reaching** 42	3-4 reps	

	Exercise	Page #	Time or reps	Exercise recommendations and variations
	Fusion sun salutation flow 2	46	3-4 reps	
	Fusion sun salutation flow 3	47	3-4 reps	
Transition	**Mountain pose.**			
Standing fusion exercises (20 min.)	**Squat**	50	8-12 reps	Move at a tempo of 2-4 counts to lower and stand up.
	Squat with heel raise	52	4-8 reps	Squat, lift the heels, lower the heels, and then stand up.
	Chair pose	54	Hold for 5 breaths.	

> continued

Exercise	Page #	Time or reps	Exercise recommendations and variations
Revolving chair	55	Hold for 5 breaths on each side.	
Single-leg squat	56	3-5 reps on each side	Move at a tempo of 2 counts to lower and stand up.
Lunge (R)	60	6-10 reps	Move at a tempo of 2-4 counts to lower and stand up.
Crescent lunge (R)	64	Hold for 3-5 breaths.	
Warrior 3 (R)	78	Hold for 3-5 breaths.	
Lunge (L)	60	6-10 reps	

Exercise	Page #	Time or reps	Exercise recommendations and variations
Crescent lunge (L)	64	Hold for 3-5 breaths.	
Warrior 3 (L)	78	Hold for 3-5 breaths.	
Warrior 1 (R)	65	Hold for 3-5 breaths.	
Warrior 2 (R)	66	Hold for 3-5 breaths.	
Reverse warrior (R)	68	Hold for 3-5 breaths.	
Extended side angle (R)	70	Hold for 3-5 breaths.	

> continued

Challenge Level Workout   > *continued*

Exercise	Page #	Time or reps	Exercise recommendations and variations
Half moon (R)	80	Hold for 3-5 breaths.	
Warrior 1 (L)	65	Hold for 3-5 breaths.	
Warrior 2 (L)	66	Hold for 3-5 breaths.	
Reverse warrior (L)	68	Hold for 3-5 breaths.	
Extended side angle (L)	70	Hold for 3-5 breaths.	
Half moon (L)	80	Hold for 3-5 breaths.	

	Exercise	Page #	Time or reps	Exercise recommendations and variations
Transition	**Perform a standing forward bend and step back to plank.**			
Floor fusion exercises (20 min.)	**Plank position**	82	Hold for 3-5 breaths.	Perform with bent knees or straight legs.
	Plank with knee tuck series	82-84	3-5 reps on each side	Alternate the leg lifts from right to left. Link the movement with the breath.
	Downward-facing dog	38	Hold for 3-5 breaths.	
	Narrow push-up	88	8-12 reps	Support weight on the knees or toes.
	Downward-facing dog	38	Hold for 3-5 breaths.	
	Side plank	90	Hold for 5 breaths on each side.	Support weight on hand or forearm.
	Two-point tabletop (R)	92	Hold for 3-5 breaths.	
	Two-point tabletop (R)	92	3-5 reps	Touch opposite knee to elbow.

> continued

Exercise	Page #	Time or reps	Exercise recommendations and variations
Two-point tabletop (L)	92	Hold for 3-5 breaths.	
Two-point tabletop (L)	92	3-5 reps	Touch opposite knee to elbow.
Back extension	94	Lift and hold for 3 breaths. Repeat 4-6 times.	Place hands at the forehead.
Hip extension	98	Lift and hold for 3 breaths. Repeat 4-6 times.	
Swimmer	95	6-8 reps each side	
Transition **Assume a tall seated position.**			
Half rollback	102	4-6 reps	Follow immediately with 4-6 reps of the oblique half rollback variation by alternating sides.
V-sit	104	Hold for 3-5 breaths.	Feet are off the floor.
Reverse table	105	Hold for 3-5 breaths.	Maintain straight legs.
Full roll-up	103	4-6 reps	Finish on your back on the floor.

Exercise	Page #	Time or reps	Exercise recommendations and variations
Side leg lift (R)	107	6-10 reps	
Side leg circle (R)	108	6-10 reps	
Side leg lift (L)	107	6-10 reps	
Side leg circle (L)	108	6-10 reps	
Abdominal brace position	112	4-6 reps	Hands can be behind the head. Lift and lower at a controlled tempo.
Bend and stretch	114	4-6 reps	
Single-leg stretch	116	6-12 reps on each side	Alternate legs.
Shoulder bridge with leg lift	119	6-10 reps on each side	Knees are bent or straight.

> continued

	Exercise	Page #	Time or reps	Exercise recommendations and variations
Calming and restorative exercises (10 min.)	**Kneeling twist (R)**	130	Hold for 5 breaths.	
	Thread the needle (R)	132	Hold for 5 breaths.	
	Kneeling twist (L)	130	Hold for 5 breaths.	
	Thread the needle (L)	132	Hold for 5 breaths.	
	Low lunge (R)	135	Hold for 5 breaths.	
	Dynamic lunge hip rock (R)	136	3-5 reps	
	Low lunge (L)	135	Hold for 5 breaths.	
	Dynamic lunge hip rock (L)	136	3-5 reps	

Exercise	Page #	Time or reps	Exercise recommendations and variations
Kneeling side bend	150	Hold for 5 breaths on each side.	
Child's pose	153	Hold for 5 breaths.	
Supported back extension	144	Hold for 5 breaths.	
Pigeon	137	Hold for 5 breaths on each side.	
Reclining butterfly	157	Hold for 5 breaths.	
Resting pose	159	Hold for 3-5 min.	Be proud of yourself for completing this workout.

9

Fusion Workouts
▮ BY TIME

The fusion workouts in this chapter are based on the amount of time you want to allocate to your workout based on your fitness level or time commitment. The shorter sessions can supplement other activities such as walking or running, or they can be done on their own as a complete workout.

Many of the warm-up exercises in chapter 4 and the calming and restorative exercises in chapter 7 can be used for either warming up or calming down. In the workout charts that follow, you will see these exercises used in either step of the workout. Refer to the page numbers for reference. The mindful exercises from chapter 3 appear in the sample workouts.

20 MINUTES

The 20-minute workout is an express workout that you can do on its own as your fusion workout for the day or combined with another activity. Use the 20-minute workout to complement your cardio workout or as a warm-up before heading out for a walk or run. You can do this efficient workout daily when your time is limited. It is also a great workout if you are a beginner because it is short and the intensity is low, making it easy to fit into your schedule. As you gain confidence and ability, progress to the longer workouts.

Intention: Even though this workout is short, focus on good execution and choose the most challenging version of each exercise when possible to give you great results in a short time.

	Exercise	Page #	Recommended time or reps	Exercise recommendations and variations
Warm-up (3 min.)	**Mountain pose with arms reaching**	42	1 min.	Center your mind and body using 3D breathing.
	Fusion sun salutation flow 2	46	3-4 reps	
Standing fusion exercises (8 min.)	**Squat**	50	8-12 reps	Move at a tempo of 2-4 counts to lower and stand up.

Exercise		Page #	Recommended time or reps	Exercise recommendations and variations
Chair pose		54	Hold for 5 deep breaths.	
Lunge (R)		60	8-12 reps	Move at a tempo of 2-4 counts to lower and stand up.
Crescent lunge (R)		64	Hold for 5 deep breaths.	
Lunge (L)		60	8-12 reps	Move at a tempo of 2-4 counts to lower and stand up.
Crescent lunge (L)		64	Hold for 5 deep breaths.	

> *continued*

	Exercise	Page #	Recommended time or reps	Exercise recommendations and variations
	Crescent lunge to warrior 3 (R)	64, 78	3-5 reps	Move from crescent lunge to warrior 3 at a controlled tempo. Hold each pose for 2-3 breaths.
	Crescent lunge to warrior 3 (L)	64, 78	3-5 reps	Move from crescent lunge to warrior 3 at a controlled tempo. Hold each pose for 2-3 breaths.
Transition				
Floor fusion exercises (6 min.)	**Plank position**	82	Hold for 5 breaths.	Support weight on hands or forearms.
	Side plank (R)	90	Hold for 5 breaths.	Support weight on hand or forearm.

	Exercise	Page #	Recommended time or reps	Exercise recommendations and variations
	Wide push-up	89	8-15 reps	Vary the tempo of the push-ups each workout: perform the push-up on a 1-count rhythm, 2-count rhythm, or 3 counts down and 1 count up.
	Side plank (L)	90	Hold for 5 breaths.	Support weight on the hand or forearm.
	Back extension	94	5 reps	Hands are on the floor or on the forehead. Lift and lower at a controlled tempo.
	Hip extension	98	5 reps	Lift and lower at a controlled tempo. Add a hold at the top of the hip extension to add intensity.
	Upward-facing dog	100	Hold for 3-5 breaths.	
	Downward-facing dog	38	Hold for 3-5 breaths.	
Transition				
Floor fusion exercises (contd.)	**Full roll-up**	103	4-8 reps	

> continued

	Exercise	Page #	Recommended time or reps	Exercise recommendations and variations
	Leg lift tabletop	113	3-5 reps on each side	Alternate legs; lift and lower at a controlled tempo.
Calming and restorative exercises (3 min.)	**Reclining single-leg hug stretch (R)**	156	Hold for 5 breaths.	
	Reclining hamstring stretch (R)	139	Hold for 5 breaths.	
	Reclining twist (R)	133	Hold for 5 breaths.	Perform with single leg.
	Reclining single-leg hug stretch (L)	156	Hold for 5 breaths.	
	Reclining hamstring stretch (L)	139	Hold for 5 breaths.	
	Reclining twist (L)	133	Hold for 5 breaths.	Perform with single leg.
	Resting pose	159	Hold for 1 min.	Although this rest is short, take full advantage of the minute. A minute of rest can make a big difference in your overall well-being.

The 40-minute fusion workout is an efficient total-body workout. This is an intermediate-level workout that will sculpt and define the entire body and focuses on strength, balance, and flexibility. Progress to this workout when the fusion begin workout is easy to complete or when you have a limited amount of time to work out. You can do this workout daily.

Intention: To get the most out of time spent, set your mind on giving this workout your full attention. When your mind wanders to other thoughts, bring yourself back to the exercises and the sensation of movement.

	Exercises	Page #	Recommended time or reps	Exercise recommendations and variations
Warm-up (5 min.)	**Mountain pose with arms reaching**	42	1 min.	Stand in mountain pose and center your mind and body using 3D breathing.
	Fusion sun salutation flow 1	45	3-4 reps	
	Fusion sun salutation flow 2	46	3-4 reps	

> continued

	Exercises	Page #	Recommended time or reps	Exercise recommendations and variations
Standing fusion exercises (15 min.)	**Curtsy squat (R)**	57	8-12 reps	Move at a tempo of 2-4 counts to lower and stand up.
	Chair pose	54	Hold for 5 deep breaths.	
	Curtsy squat (L)	57	8-12 reps	Move at a tempo of 2-4 counts to lower and stand up.
	Lunge to single-leg balance (R)	60, 72	8-10 reps	Stand with weight equally on both feet and step the right leg back into the lunge at a tempo of 2-4 counts to lower. Stand up bringing the right knee up into a knee balance. Repeat.
	Revolving chair (R)	55	Hold for 5 breaths.	

	Exercises	Page #	Recommended time or reps	Exercise recommendations and variations
	Lunge to single-leg balance (L)	60, 72	8-10 reps	
	Revolving chair (L)	55	Hold for 5 breaths.	
Transition				
Floor fusion exercises (15 min.)	**Half rollback**	102	4-6 reps	Follow immediately with 4-6 reps of the oblique half rollback variation by alternating sides.
	Full roll-up	103	4-6 reps	
	Abdominal brace position	112	4-6 reps	Hands can be behind the head. Curl up and hold for 3-4 breaths. On each exhalation, increase the abdominal tension.
	Leg lift tabletop	113	5-10 reps on each side	Alternate leg lifts and lower at a controlled tempo.

> continued

	Exercises	Page #	Recommended time or reps	Exercise recommendations and variations
	Bend and stretch	114	4-8 reps	
	Single-leg stretch	116	5-10 reps on each side	
	Shoulder bridge with leg lift	119	Hold for 5 breaths on each side.	Perform with bent knee or straight leg.
	Side bend	109	3-5 reps on each side	
Transition				
Calming and restorative exercises (5 min.)	**Kneeling twist (R)**	130	Hold for 3 breaths.	
	Thread the needle (R)	132	Hold for 3 breaths.	

Exercises	Page #	Recommended time or reps	Exercise recommendations and variations
Kneeling twist (L)	130	Hold for 3 breaths.	
Thread the needle (L)	132	Hold for 3 breaths.	
Low lunge (R)	135	Hold for 3-5 breaths.	
Revolving lunge (R)	62	Hold for 3-5 breaths.	
Puppy pose	126	Hold for 3 breaths.	
Low lunge (L)	135	Hold for 3-5 breaths.	
Revolving lunge (L)	62	Hold for 3-5 breaths.	
Child's pose	153	Hold for 1 min.	

60 MINUTES

The 60-minute fusion workout is a challenging total-body workout. This workout targets all of the major muscles of the body and trains strength, balance, and flexibility. Progress from the shorter and easier workouts to this full-body sculpting workout. Choose the exercise intensity that is best for you, and refer to the exercises in chapters 4 through 7 for options and variations. As you master this workout, you can add intensity by doing more repetitions of each exercise or longer holds.

Intention: Focus your mind on being strong and determined.

	Exercise	Page #	Recommended time or reps	Exercise recommendations and variations
Warm-up (8 min.)	**Mountain pose with arms reaching**	42	1 min.	Stand in mountain pose and center your mind and body using 3D breathing.
	Fusion sun salutation flow 1	45	2-3 reps	
	Fusion sun salutation flow 2	46	2-3 reps	

	Exercise	Page #	Recommended time or reps	Exercise recommendations and variations
	Fusion sun salutation flow 3	47	2-3 reps	
Standing fusion exercises (20 min.)	**Single-leg squat (R)**	56	8-12 reps	
	Single-leg squat (L)	56	8-12 reps	
	Lunge (R)	60	8-12 reps	Step back to the lunge from mountain pose at a tempo of 2-4 counts to lower, and step back to mountain pose.
	Crescent lunge (R)	64	Hold for 3-5 breaths.	Step back and stay in the lunge to move to crescent lunge.
	Warrior 3 (R)	78	Hold for 3-5 breaths.	Lift up to balance from crescent lunge to warrior 3.

> continued

Exercise	Page #	Recommended time or reps	Exercise recommendations and variations
Single-leg balance (R) 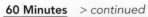	72	Hold for 3-5 breaths.	Stay on the same leg for single-leg balance.
Squat with heel raise	52	8-12 reps	Lower and lift on a 2-count rhythm.
Lunge (L)	60	8-10 reps	Step back to the lunge from mountain pose at a tempo of 2-4 counts to lower, and step back to mountain pose.
Crescent lunge (L)	64	Hold for 3-5 breaths.	Step back and stay in the lunge to move to crescent lunge.
Warrior 3 (L)	78	Hold for 3-5 breaths.	Lift up to balance from crescent lunge to warrior 3.
Single-leg balance (L)	72	Hold for 3-5 breaths.	Stay on the same leg for single-leg balance.

	Exercise	Page #	Recommended time or reps	Exercise recommendations and variations
	Curtsy squat (R)	57	8-12 reps	Perform the variation with rotation. Lower and lift on a 2-count rhythm.
	Half moon (R)	80	Hold for 3-5 breaths.	
	Curtsy squat (L)	57	8-12 reps	Perform the variation with rotation. Lower and lift on a 2-count rhythm.
	Half moon (L)	80	Hold for 3-5 breaths.	
Transition	**Perform a standing forward bend and step back to plank.**			
Floor fusion exercises (25 min.)	**Plank position**	82	Hold for 3-5 breaths.	
	Plank to hip drop	87	6-8 reps on each side	
	Child's pose	153	Hold for 3 breaths.	

> continued

Exercise	Page #	Recommended time or reps	Exercise recommendations and variations
Wide push-up	89	8-12 reps	
Back extension	94	4-6 reps	Arms can be extended overhead.
Hip extension	98	4-6 reps	Perform the bend-and-straighten variation.
Upward-facing dog	100	Hold for 3 breaths.	
Side plank (R)	90	Hold for 3 breaths.	Support weight on the forearm or hand.
Side leg circle (R)	108	4-6 reps	Support weight on the forearm or hand.
Side bend (R)	109	4-6 reps	
Breaststroke	96	4-6 reps	
Side plank (L)	90	Hold for 3 breaths.	Support weight on the forearm or hand.

Exercise	Page #	Recommended time or reps	Exercise recommendations and variations
Side leg circle (L)	108	4-6 reps	Support weight on the forearm or hand.
Side bend (L)	109	4-6 reps	
Knee-tuck series	84	3-5 reps	
V-sit	104	Hold for 5 breaths.	
Reverse table	105	Hold for 5 breaths.	
Full roll-up	103	3-5 reps	
Leg lift tabletop	113	4-6 reps on each side	
Single-leg stretch	116	5-10 reps on each side	
Crisscross	117	5-10 reps on each side	

> continued

	Exercise	Page #	Recommended time or reps	Exercise recommendations and variations
	Shoulder bridge with leg lift	119	5-10 reps on each side	Lift and lower on a 2-count rhythm. Leg is lifted in a bent or straight position.
Calming and restorative exercises (7 min.)	**Reclining knee-hug stretch**	155	Hold for 3-5 breaths.	
	Reclining single-leg hug stretch (R)	156	Hold for 3-5 breaths.	
	Reclining hamstring stretch (R)	139	Hold for 3-5 breaths.	
	Reclining figure-4 (R)	142	Hold for 3-5 breaths.	
	Reclining single-leg hug stretch (L)	156	Hold for 3-5 breaths.	
	Reclining hamstring stretch (L)	139	Hold for 3-5 breaths.	

Exercise	Page #	Recommended time or reps	Exercise recommendations and variations
Reclining figure-4 (L)	142	Hold for 3-5 breaths.	
Seated forward bend	123	Hold for 3-5 breaths.	
Seated butterfly	138	Hold for 3-5 breaths.	
Cross-legged seated twist	129	Hold for 3-5 breaths on each side.	
Cross-legged seated forward bend	125	Hold for 3-5 breaths on each side.	
Seated simple meditation		3-5 min.	Find a comfortable seated position. Close your eyes and calm your breathing. Reflect on the workout you have completed and allow yourself a moment of gratitude.

10

Fusion Workouts
▌BY PURPOSE

The fusion workouts in this chapter are based on your purpose for training. The exercises are grouped to produce the best results for the specific focus of your workout. Choose one workout by itself, or mix the workouts in this section to give you a variety of options. For example, do just the core conditioning workout, or do the core conditioning workout followed by upper-body conditioning. You can also do one of the fusion workouts in this section to complement your cardio workout. Many of the warm-up exercises in chapter 4 and the calming and restorative exercises in chapter 7 can be used for either warming up or calming down. In the workout charts that follow, you will see these exercises used in either step of the workout. Refer to the page numbers for reference. The mindful exercises from chapter 3 appear in the sample workouts.

CORE CONDITIONING WORKOUT

Strengthening the core muscles improves posture, increases performance of any activity, protects the back, and defines the muscles of the core. You can gain the benefits of core training by adding this workout to your regular routine. The core conditioning workout is based on the most current core conditioning methods using a three-dimensional approach to training the core for the best results. Traditional core strengthening exercises, such as an abdominal crunch, are performed in one direction, flexion, and are less effective in training the core. Exercises that take the body through multiple planes of movement and a variety of body positions where the spine flexes, extends, rotates, and bends are far more effective. The core muscles work to move you and stabilize against gravity. By performing exercises where the core has to work to hold a body position against gravity increase your ability to stabilize the spine, hips, and shoulders. The exercises in the fusion core conditioning workout are integrated and will work the core in the way it is meant to be trained: as a mover and a stabilizer.

Start by doing the core workout twice a week and work up to five times per week. Refer to the exercise library in chapters 4 through 7 for exercise modifications and variations.

Intention: Focus on using your 3D breathing technique to activate the deep core muscles throughout this workout.

	Exercise	Page #	Recommended time or reps	Exercise recommendations and variations
Warm-up (5 min.)	Seated 3D breathing	13	1-2 min.	Sit in a comfortable position and center your mind and body with deep breathing.
	Child's pose	29	Hold for 3-5 breaths.	Focus on stretching through the shoulders and lengthening along the spine from the shoulders to the tailbone.
	Cat and cow stretch	30	3-5 reps	

	Exercise	Page #	Recommended time or reps	Exercise recommendations and variations
	Spinal rotation with thread the needle	30	3-5 reps on each side	
	Plank to narrow push-up to upward-facing dog to downward-facing dog	82, 88, 100, 38	3-5 reps	Flow from each of the exercises with 1-2 breaths.
Transition	From downward-facing dog, step forward into the lunge.			
Standing fusion exercises (20 min.)	**Lunge to warrior 3 (R)**	60, 78	8-12 reps	Flow dynamically from lunge to warrior 3 with 1-2 breaths per exercise.

> continued

Exercise	Page #	Recommended time or reps	Exercise recommendations and variations
Lunge to warrior 3 (L)	60, 78	8-12 reps	Flow dynamically from lunge to warrior 3 with 1-2 breaths per exercise.
Single-leg squat (R)	56	8-12 reps	Flow from single-leg squat to curtsy squat.
Curtsy squat (R)	57	8-12 reps	Flow from curtsy squat to curtsy squat with rotation. Complete 8-12 reps in both variations.
Single-leg squat (L)	56	8-12 reps	Flow from single-leg squat to curtsy squat.
Curtsy squat (L)	57	8-12 reps	Flow from curtsy squat to curtsy squat with rotation. Complete 8-12 reps in both variations.

Exercise	Page #	Recommended time or reps	Exercise recommendations and variations
Single-leg balance (R)	72	Hold for 3-5 breaths.	
Side balance (R)	74	Hold for 3-5 breaths.	
Ballet squat with heel raise	59	4-6 reps	
Single-leg balance (L)	72	Hold for 3-5 breaths.	
Side balance (L)	74	Hold for 3-5 breaths.	

> continued

	Exercise	Page #	Recommended time or reps	Exercise recommendations and variations
	Half moon	80	Hold for 3-5 breaths on each side.	
Transition	**Perform a standing forward bend and step back to a kneeling position.**			
Floor fusion exercises (25 min.)	**Two-point tabletop**	92	3-5 reps of each exercise variation per side	Alternate the arm and leg lift, reach opposite knee to elbow, and then do the leg-crossover variation.
	Plank position	82	Hold for 3-5 breaths.	
	Plank with leg lift	83	6-8 reps on each side	
	Narrow push-up	88	6-10 reps	
	Child's pose	153	Hold for 3-5 breaths.	
	Knee-tuck series	84	3-5 reps each side	
	Child's pose	153	Hold for 3-5 breaths.	

Exercise		Page #	Recommended time or reps	Exercise recommendations and variations
Side plank (R)		90	Hold for 3-5 breaths.	Support weight on forearm or hand.
Side bend (R)		109	3-5 reps	Support weight on forearm or hand.
Side twist (R)		110	3-5 reps	Support weight on forearm or hand.
Plank with hip drive		86	3-5 reps each side	
Side plank (L)		90	Hold for 3-5 breaths.	Support weight on forearm or hand.
Side bend (L)		109	3-5 reps	Support weight on forearm or hand.
Side twist (L)		110	3-5 reps	Support weight on forearm or hand.

> continued

Exercise	Page #	Recommended time or reps	Exercise recommendations and variations
Wide push-up	89	8-12 reps	
Childs pose	153	Hold for 3-5 breaths.	
Swimmer	95	8 to 10 reps	
Breaststroke	96	3-5 reps	
Plank to hip drop	87	3-5 reps on each side	
V-sit	104	Hold for 3-5 breaths.	
Reverse table	105	Hold for 3-5 breaths.	
Half rollback	102	4-6 reps	
Half rollback	102	4-6 reps on each side	Perform oblique variation.

Exercise	Page #	Recommended time or reps	Exercise recommendations and variations
Full roll-up	103	4-6 reps	
Abdominal brace position	112	3-5 reps	Hands can be behind the head. Curl up and hold for 1-2 breaths, then lower.
Leg lift tabletop	113	6-10 reps	
Single-leg stretch	116	6-10 reps on each side	
Crisscross	117	6-10 reps on each side	
Bend and stretch	114	6-10 reps	
Shoulder bridge with leg lift	119	Hold for 5 breaths on each side.	Perform bent or straight-leg option.

> continued

Core Conditioning Workout > continued

	Exercise	Page #	Recommended time or reps	Exercise recommendations and variations
Calming and restorative exercises (5 min.)	Kneeling twist	130	Hold for 3-5 breaths on each side.	Perform with both legs.
	Low lunge (R)	135	Hold for 3-5 breaths.	
	Dynamic lunge hip rock (R)	136	Hold for 3-5 breaths.	
	Pigeon (R)	137	Hold for 3-5 breaths.	
	Low lunge (L)	135	Hold for 3-5 breaths.	
	Dynamic lunge hip rock (L)	136	Hold for 3-5 breaths.	
	Pigeon (L)	137	Hold for 3-5 breaths.	

Exercise	Page #	Recommended time or reps	Exercise recommendations and variations
Kneeling side bend	150	Hold for 3-5 breaths on each side.	
Reclining knee-hug stretch	155	Hold for 5 breaths.	
Reclining twist	133	Hold for 5 breaths on each side.	
Reclining butterfly	157	Hold for 5 breaths.	
Resting pose	159	3-5 min.	Practice positive self-talk. While you rest, list in your mind all of the things you do well.

FULL-BODY CONDITIONING WORKOUT

The name of this workout says it all. This is a full-body conditioning workout that targets the upper body, core, and lower body. In this complete workout you can select the easier or more challenging options from the fusion exercises in chapters 4 through 7. This is a great workout when you want to accomplish a lot in one training session. You can do this workout three to five times per week. As you gain strength and skill, add more repetitions or hold the exercises longer.

Intention: Approach this workout with a positive attitude. Focus on your strengths and know you will get stronger with practice.

	Exercise	Page #	Recommended time or reps	Exercise recommendations and variations
Warm-up (10 mins.)	**Standing 3D breathing**	13	1 min.	Stand and center your mind and body with deep breathing.
	Mountain pose with arms reaching	42	3-4 reps	
	Mountain pose with side bend	43	3-4 reps on each side	
	Dynamic four-point stretch	146	3-4 reps	Move at a controlled pace.

	Exercise	Page #	Recommended time or reps	Exercise recommendations and variations
	Standing forward bend	41	Hold for 3-5 breaths.	Curve the spine and roll down and up in a slow, controlled manner.
	Fusion sun salutation flow 2	46	3-5 reps	
	Fusion sun salutation flow 3	47	3-5 reps	
Transition	**Come to mountain pose.**			
Standing fusion exercises (15 min.)	**Lunge (R)**	60	8-12 reps	From mountain pose, step back and together.
	Crescent lunge (R)	64	Hold for 3-5 breaths.	From crescent lunge, lift the back leg up to warrior 3.

> continued

Exercise	Page #	Recommended time or reps	Exercise recommendations and variations
Warrior 3 (R)	78	Hold for 3-5 breaths.	
Lunge (L)	60	8-10 reps	From warrior 3, step back and together.
Crescent lunge (L)	64	Hold for 3-5 breaths.	From crescent lunge, lift the back leg up to warrior 3.
Warrior 3 (L)	78	Hold for 3-5 breaths.	
Squat	50	8-10 reps	Lower and stand up on a 2- or 4-count rhythm.
Revolving chair	55	Hold for 3-5 breaths on each side.	

Exercise	Page #	Recommended time or reps	Exercise recommendations and variations
Single-leg balance (R)	72	Hold for 3-5 breaths.	
Single-leg squat (R)	56	8-10 reps	
Single-leg balance (L)	72	Hold for 3-5 breaths.	
Single-leg squat (L)	56	8-10 reps	
Ballet squat	58	8-10 reps	
Ballet squat with heel raise	59	8-10 reps	

> continued

	Exercise	Page #	Recommended time or reps	Exercise recommendations and variations
	Tree pose	76	Hold for 5 breaths on each side.	
Transition	Perform a standing forward bend and step back to plank.			
Floor fusion exercises (20 min.)	**Plank position**	82	Hold for 3-5 breaths.	
	Plank with hip drive	86	4-8 reps	
	Wide push-up	89	8-10 reps	Support weight on knees or toes
	Side plank (R)	90	Hold for 3-5 breaths.	Support weight on forearm or hand.
	Swimmer	95	8-10 reps	
	Side plank (L)	90	Hold for 3-5 breaths.	Support weight on forearm or hand.

Exercise	Page #	Recommended time or reps	Exercise recommendations and variations
Upward-facing dog	100	Hold for 3-5 breaths.	
Dynamic bow	99	3-5 reps	
Side bend to side twist (R)	109, 110	3-5 reps	
V-sit	104	Hold for 3-5 breaths.	
Side bend to side twist (L)	109, 110	3-5 reps	
Half rollback	102	4-8 reps	

> continued

Full-Body Conditioning Workout > *continued*

	Exercise	Page #	Recommended time or reps	Exercise recommendations and variations
	Full roll-up	103	3-5 reps	
	Leg lift tabletop	113	8-10 reps	
	Shoulder bridge in external rotation	120	8-10 reps	Lift and lower on a 2-count rhythm.
Transition	**Come to a seated position.**			
Calming and restorative exercises (10 mins.)	**Cross-legged seated forward bend**	125	Hold for 3-5 breaths on each side.	
	Seated twist	128	Hold for 3-5 breaths on each side.	
	Seated cow face pose	145	Hold for 3-5 breaths on each side.	
	Seated side bend	149	Hold for 3-5 breaths on each side.	
	Wide-legged forward bend	124	Hold for 3-5 breaths.	

Exercise	Page #	Recommended time or reps	Exercise recommendations and variations
Dynamic lunge hip rock	136	3-5 reps on each side	
Revolving lunge	62	Hold for 3-5 breaths on each side.	
Supported back extension	144	Hold for 3-5 breaths.	
Child's pose	153	Hold for 3-5 breaths.	
Seated simple meditation		2-5 min.	Bring your awareness to your breath. Observe the subtle movements of your body during each inhalation and exhalation. If the mind wanders, bring it back to your breath.

UPPER-BODY CONDITIONING WORKOUT

The use of modern conveniences and technology in everyday life has changed the way we use the upper body. Previous generations worked the upper body during everyday chores. For most people, this is no longer the case, so weakness in the upper body results. Training the upper body is vital for overall fitness, function, and appearance. The fusion upper-body conditioning workout targets all of the major muscle groups of the upper body without using weights or other fitness equipment. The organization of the workout will give you an upper-body challenge that defines the arms, chest, and back while integrating core conditioning. The upper-body conditioning workout is a great supplement to other activities such as walking and running. Depending on your weekly fusion workout program, you could do this workout three times per week. Make adjustments to the exercises in chapters 4 through 7 to make the workout harder or easier and adjust the number of repetitions or exercise variation.

Intention: This is a challenging workout. Give it your best effort and know that in time you will get stronger. Focus on the mantra *I am strong.*

	Exercise	Page #	Recommended time or reps.	Exercise descriptions, recommendations, and variations
Warm-up (8 min.)	**Standing 3D breathing**	13	1-2 min.	Stand and center your mind and body with deep breathing.
	Mountain pose with arms reaching	42	3-4 reps	
	Mountain pose with side bend	43	3-4 reps on each side	

Exercise	Page #	Recommended time or reps.	Exercise descriptions, recommendations, and variations
Dynamic four-point stretch	146	3-5 reps	Move at a controlled pace.
Fusion sun salutation flow 2	46	3-5 reps	
Fusion sun salutation flow 3	47	3-5 reps	

Transition	**Come to mountain pose.**			
Standing fusion exercises (10 min.)	**Warrior 1 (R)**	65	Hold for 3-5 breaths.	
	Warrior 2 (R)	66	Hold for 3-5 breaths.	

> continued

Exercise	Page #	Recommended time or reps.	Exercise descriptions, recommendations, and variations
Reverse warrior (R)	68	Hold for 3-5 breaths.	
Extended side angle (R)	70	Hold for 3-5 breaths.	
Crescent lunge (R)	64	Hold for 3-5 breaths.	
Plank to narrow push-up to upward-facing dog to downward-facing dog	82, 88, 100, 38	Flow through each of the exercises at a controlled pace, 1-2 deep breaths per movement.	From the crescent lunge, bring the hands to the floor and step back into plank. Step into warrior 1 from downward-facing dog.

Exercise	Page #	Recommended time or reps.	Exercise descriptions, recommendations, and variations
Warrior 1 (L)	65	Hold for 3-5 breaths.	
Warrior 2 (L)	66	Hold for 3-5 breaths.	
Reverse Warrior (L)	68	Hold for 3-5 breaths.	
Extended side angle (L)	70	Hold for 3-5 breaths.	
Crescent lunge (L)	64	Hold for 3-5 breaths.	

> continued

	Exercise	Page #	Recommended time or reps.	Exercise descriptions, recommendations, and variations
	Plank to narrow push-up to upward-facing dog to downward-facing dog	82, 88, 100, 38	Flow through each of the exercises at a controlled pace, 1-2 deep breaths per movement.	From the crescent lunge, bring the hands to the floor and step back into plank.
Transition	**Lower to the knees from downward-facing dog.**			
Floor fusion exercises (25 min.)	**Plank position**	82	Hold for 5-10 breaths.	Support weight on knees or toes.
	Narrow push-up	88	8-10 reps	Support weight on knees or toes.
	Child's pose	29	Hold for 3-5 breaths.	Use this exercise to rest.
	Plank position	37	Hold for 3-5 breaths.	Lift right leg and support weight on knees or toes.
	Narrow push-up	88	8-10 reps	Lift right leg and support weight on knees or toes.
	Child's pose	29	Hold for 3-5 breaths.	Use this exercise to rest.
	Plank position	82	Hold for 3-5 breaths.	Lift left leg and support weight on knees or toes.

Exercise	Page #	Recommended time or reps.	Exercise descriptions, recommendations, and variations
Narrow push-up	88	8-10 reps	Lift left leg and support weight on knees or toes.
Back extension	94	8-10 reps	Perform with arms reaching out to the side.
Breaststroke	96	3-5 reps	
Side plank (R)	90	Hold for 3-5 breaths.	Support weight on hand or forearm.
Wide push-up	89	8-10 reps	Support weight on knees or toes.
Side plank (L)	90	Hold for 3-5 breaths.	Support weight on hand or forearm.
Swimmer	95	8-10 reps	
Upward-facing dog	100	Hold for 3-5 breaths.	
Side bend (R)	109	3-5 reps	

> continued

	Exercise	Page #	Recommended time or reps.	Exercise descriptions, recommendations, and variations
	Side twist (R)	110		
	Reverse table	105	Hold for 3-5 breaths.	Perform exercise with bent knees or straight legs.
	Side bend (L)	109	3-5 reps	
	Side twist (L)	110	3-5 reps	
Transition	Stay in a seated position.			
Calming and restorative exercises (8 min.)	Seated cow face pose	145	Hold for 3-5 breaths on each side.	
	Seated twist	128	Hold for 3-5 breaths on each side.	
	Seated side bend	149	Hold for 3-5 breaths on each side.	
	Seated forward bend	123	Hold for 3-5 breaths.	

Exercise	Page #	Recommended time or reps.	Exercise descriptions, recommendations, and variations
Reclining twist	133	Hold for 3-5 breaths on each side.	Both legs are bent.
Resting pose	159	1-5 min.	Take time to restore the body, slow the heart rate and breathing rate, and to become calm.

LOWER-BODY CONDITIONING WORKOUT

The lower-body conditioning workout targets the hips, buttocks, and thighs. The exercises in this workout will strengthen and define the lower body, while at the same time increase flexibility and stability to achieve movement that is powerful and graceful. The lower-body workout can be done two to four times per week depending on your total weekly fusion workouts. Increase the workout by adding more repetitions or hold the exercises longer.

Intention: Focus on finding equilibrium in your body. Observe whether one side of the body is stronger, more stable, or more flexible. Spend more time on the weaknesses that you observe.

	Exercise	Page #	Recommended time or reps	Exercise descriptions, recommendations, and variations
Warm-up (5 min.)	**Standing 3D breathing**	13	1 min.	Stand and center your mind and body through deep breathing.
	Mountain pose with arms reaching	42	3-4 reps	
	Mountain pose with side bend	43	3-4 reps on each side	
	Standing forward bend	41	Hold for 3-5 breaths.	

	Exercise	Page #	Recommended time or reps	Exercise descriptions, recommendations, and variations
	Fusion sun salutation flow 2	46	3-5 reps	
	Low lunge to kneeling hamstring stretch	34	3-5 reps on each side	
Transition	**Mountain pose.**			
Standing fusion exercises (20 min.)	**Squat**	50	8-12 reps	Lower and stand up on a 2-count rhythm.
	Squat with heel raise	52	8-12 reps	
	Single-leg squat (R)	56	8-10 reps	

> continued

Exercise	Page #	Recommended time or reps	Exercise descriptions, recommendations, and variations
Single-leg squat (L)	56	8-10 reps	
Warrior 1 (R)	65	Hold for 3-5 breaths.	
Warrior 2 (R)	66	Hold for 3-5 breaths.	
Reverse warrior (R)	68	Hold for 3-5 breaths.	
Extended side angle (R)	70	Hold for 3-5 breaths.	
Warrior 1 (L)	65	Hold for 3-5 breaths.	

Exercise	Page #	Recommended time or reps	Exercise descriptions, recommendations, and variations
Warrior 2 (L)	66	Hold for 3-5 breaths.	
Reverse warrior (L)	68	Hold for 3-5 breaths.	
Extended side angle (L)	70	Hold for 3-5 breaths.	
Lunge (R)	60	8-12 reps	Lower and stand up on a 2-count rhythm.
Crescent lunge (R)	64	Hold for 3-5 breaths.	
Revolving lunge (R)	62	Hold for 3-5 breaths.	

> continued

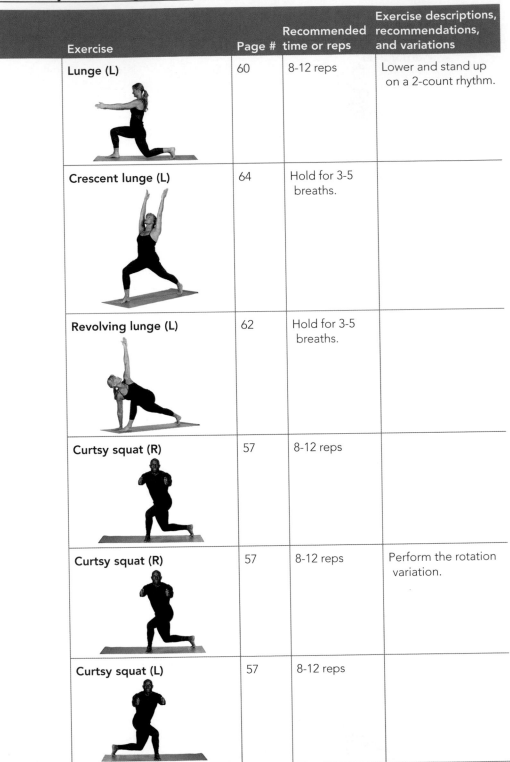

Exercise	Page #	Recommended time or reps	Exercise descriptions, recommendations, and variations
Lunge (L)	60	8-12 reps	Lower and stand up on a 2-count rhythm.
Crescent lunge (L)	64	Hold for 3-5 breaths.	
Revolving lunge (L)	62	Hold for 3-5 breaths.	
Curtsy squat (R)	57	8-12 reps	
Curtsy squat (R)	57	8-12 reps	Perform the rotation variation.
Curtsy squat (L)	57	8-12 reps	

Exercise	Page #	Recommended time or reps	Exercise descriptions, recommendations, and variations
Curtsy squat (L)	57	8-12 reps	Perform the rotation variation.
Chair pose	54	Hold for 5 breaths.	
Revolving chair	55	Hold for 3-5 breaths on each side.	
Ballet squat	58	8-12 reps	
Ballet squat with heel raise	59	8-12 reps	

Transition	Perform a standing forward bend and step back to a kneeling position			
Floor fusion exercises (25 min.)	Two-point tabletop	92	3-5 reps on each side	Alternate arm and leg lift.

> continued

Exercise	Page #	Recommended time or reps	Exercise descriptions, recommendations, and variations
Two-point table top	92	3-5 reps on each side	Perform leg cross-over.
Hip extension	92	Hold for 3-5 breaths and repeat 3 times.	Perform with straight leg.
Hip extension	98	8-10 reps	Bend and straighten.
Side leg lift (R)	107	8-10 reps	
Side leg circle (R)	108	8-10 reps	Support weight on hand or forearm.
Side bend (R)	109	3-5 reps	
Side leg lift (L)	107	8-10 reps	
Side leg circle (L)	108	8-10 reps	Support weight on hand or forearm.
Side bend (L)	109	3-5 reps	
Reverse table	105	Hold for 3-5 breaths and repeat 3 times.	Perform with bent knees or straight legs.

	Exercise	Page #	Recommended time or reps	Exercise descriptions, recommendations, and variations
	Shoulder bridge	118	8-10 reps	Lift and lower on a 2-count rhythm.
	Shoulder bridge in external rotation	120	8-10 reps	Lift and lower on a 2-count rhythm.
Transition	**Come to a kneeling position.**			
Calming and restorative exercises (10 min.)	**Low lunge (R)**	135	Hold for 3-5 breaths.	
	Dynamic lunge hip rock (R)	136	3-5 reps	
	Pigeon (R)	137	Hold for 3-5 breaths.	
	Low lunge (L)	135	Hold for 3-5 breaths.	
	Dynamic lunge hip rock (L)	136	3-5 reps	
	Pigeon (L)	137	Hold for 3-5 breaths.	

> continued

Lower-Body Conditioning Workout   > *continued*

Exercise	Page #	Recommended time or reps	Exercise descriptions, recommendations, and variations
Reclining single-leg hug stretch	156	Hold for 3-5 breaths on each side.	
Reclining hamstring stretch	139	Hold for 3-5 breaths on each side.	
Reclining adductor stretch	140	Hold for 3-5 breaths on each side.	
Reclining abductor stretch	141	Hold for 3-5 breaths on each side.	
Reclining figure-4	142	Hold for 3-5 breaths on each side.	
Happy baby	158	Hold for 3-5 breaths.	
Reclining butterfly	157	1 min.	Breathe and relax.

RESTORATION AND RELAXATION WORKOUT

This workout is designed to calm and restore the body. Complete this workout on days when you simply need to relax more than you need to work hard. As you plan your weekly workouts, schedule the restoration and relaxation workout the day after a high-intensity workout to help the body recover. You can also do this workout after another activity as a great way to stretch and relax. You can do the fusion restoration and relaxation workout daily.

Intention: This workout is all about letting go. Surrender yourself to the exercises and stretches in this workout. Observe your breath, and keep it slow and relaxed.

	Exercise	Page #	Recommended time or reps	Exercise descriptions, recommendations, and variations
Warm-up (5-15 min.)	Seated 3D breathing	13	1 min.	Sit and center your mind and body through deep breathing.
	Seated positive-thoughts meditation		3-10 min.	You can set a timer for this section to allow your mind to rest into your meditation. Focus on a positive thought or phrase that brings you joy and peace.
	Child's pose	29	Hold for 5-10 breaths.	Puppy pose is an option if child's pose is not comfortable.
	Cat and cow stretch	30	3-5 reps	
Transition	**Come to a seated position.**			
Calming and restorative exercises (20-30 min.)	Cross-legged seated forward bend	125	Hold for 5 breaths on each side.	

> continued

Exercise	Page #	Recommended time or reps	Exercise descriptions, recommendations, and variations
Seated side bend	149	Hold for 5 breaths on each side.	
Seated twist	128	Hold for 5 breaths on each side.	
Seated forward bend	123	Hold for 5 breaths.	
Seated butterfly	138	Hold for 5 breaths.	
Seated cow face pose	145	Hold for 5 breaths on each side.	
Wide-legged forward bend	124	Hold for 5 breaths.	
Low lunge (R)	135	Hold for 5 breaths.	
Revolving lunge (R)	62	Hold for 5 breaths.	

Exercise	Page #	Recommended time or reps	Exercise descriptions, recommendations, and variations
Pigeon (R)	137	Hold for 5 breaths.	
Puppy pose	126	Hold for 5 breaths.	
Low lunge (L)	135	Hold for 5 breaths.	
Revolving lunge (L)	62	Hold for 5 breaths.	
Pigeon (L)	137	Hold for 5 breaths.	
Kneeling twist	130	Hold for 5 breaths on each side.	
Supported back extension	144	Hold for 5 breaths.	
Child's pose	153	Hold for 5 breaths.	

> continued

Exercise	Page #	Recommended time or reps	Exercise descriptions, recommendations, and variations
Reclining knee-hug stretch	155	Hold for 5 breaths.	
Reclining single-leg hug stretch (R)	156	Hold for 5 breaths.	Perform with knee circle.
Reclining hamstring stretch (R)	139	Hold for 5 breaths.	
Reclining abductor stretch (R)	141	Hold for 5 breaths.	
Reclining adductor stretch (R)	140	Hold for 5 breaths.	
Reclining figure-4 (R)	142	Hold for 5 breaths.	
Reclining twist (R)	133	Hold for 5 breaths.	
Reclining knee-hug stretch	155	Hold for 5 breaths.	

Exercise	Page #	Recommended time or reps	Exercise descriptions, recommendations, and variations
Reclining single-leg hug stretch (L)	156	Hold for 5 breaths.	Perform with knee circle.
Reclining hamstring stretch (L)	139	Hold for 5 breaths.	
Reclining abductor stretch (L)	141	Hold for 5 breaths.	
Reclining adductor stretch (L)	140	Hold for 5 breaths.	
Reclining figure-4 (L)	142	Hold for 5 breaths.	
Reclining twist (L)	133	Hold for 5 breaths.	
Reclining butterfly	157	Hold for 5 breaths.	
Happy baby	158	Hold for 5 breaths.	

> continued

Restoration and Relaxation Workout   > continued

Exercise	Page #	Recommended time or reps	Exercise descriptions, recommendations, and variations
Calm lake	154	Hold for 5 breaths.	
Resting pose	159	1-10 min.	Bring your focus to your breath. Allow your inhalation and exhalation to become slow and calm until you breathe without effort.

Fusion Workouts

▌ BY ACTIVITY

The workouts and exercises in this chapter are based on the activity and the style of workout you want to experience. Practice a workout based on the Pilates and fitness exercises to give you a strong core workout, or perform the exercises in the barre category to challenge balance, flexibility, and grace. By varying the number of repetitions or the duration of the exercises, you can easily increase or decrease your workout intensity. Many of the warm-up exercises in chapter 4 and the calming and restorative exercises in chapter 7 can be used for either warming up or calming down. In the workout charts that follow, you will see these exercises used in either step of the workout. Refer to the page numbers for reference. The mindful exercises from chapter 3 appear in the sample workouts.

ATHLETE WORKOUT

Whether you are a fitness enthusiast or a recreational or competitive athlete, training can cause tension and create muscle imbalances. The most common result of fitness activities is a tightening of the hips, low back, front of the shoulders, and chest. The exercises in this workout aim to release tension and increase mobility in these trouble areas and at the same time build strength. The athlete workout is physical and challenging. You can do this workout three times per week and should supplement it with easier workouts such as the 20-minute workout and the restoration and relaxation workout. Vary the number of repetitions and length of the holds to increase or decrease the intensity of this workout.

Intention: It is time to let go of competitiveness with yourself or others. Be aware of pushing too hard. Become aware of what you feel, and respect your limitations.

	Exercise	Page #	Recommended time or reps	Exercise descriptions, recommendations, and variations
Warm-up (10 min.)	**Child's pose**	29	Hold for 5 breaths	Practice 3D breathing and focus on expanding the back of the rib cage.
	Cat and cow stretch	30	3-4 reps	Move from cat to cow at a controlled pace.
	Spinal rotation with thread the needle	32	3-4 reps on each side	Move from spinal rotation to thread the needle in 2-3 breaths per movement.

Exercise	Page #	Recommended time or reps	Exercise descriptions, recommendations, and variations
Low lunge to kneeling hamstring stretch	34	3-4 reps on each side	Move from the lunge with the hands on the floor to the hamstring stretch at a controlled tempo.
Downward-facing dog	38	Hold for 5 breaths.	If downward-facing dog is uncomfortable, do child's pose.
Standing forward bend	41	3-4 reps	Curve the spine and roll down and up at a slow controlled rhythm.
Fusion sun salutation flow 1	45	2-3 reps	
Fusion sun salutation flow 2	46	2-3 reps	

> continued

	Exercise	Page #	Recommended time or reps	Exercise descriptions, recommendations, and variations
Transition	From standing or from downward-facing dog, step into a lunge.			
Standing fusion exercises (15 min.)	**Crescent lunge (R)**	64	Hold for 3-5 breaths.	Arms are overhead. A variation is to keep the arms behind the back.
	Lunge (R)	60	Hold for 3-5 breaths.	Hands are on the floor.
	Revolving lunge (R)	62	Hold for 3-5 breaths.	
	Downward-facing dog	38	Hold for 3-5 breaths.	
	Crescent lunge (L)	64	Hold for 3-5 breaths.	Arms are overhead. A variation is to keep the arms behind the back.
	Lunge (L)	60	Hold for 3-5 breaths.	Hands are on the floor.

Exercise	Page #	Recommended time or reps	Exercise descriptions, recommendations, and variations
Revolving lunge (L)	62	Hold for 3-5 breaths.	
Warrior 2 (R)	67	Hold for 3-5 breaths.	
Reverse warrior (R)	68	Hold for 3-5 breaths.	
Extended side angle (R)	70	Hold for 3-5 breaths.	
Half moon (R)	80	Hold for 3-5 breaths.	
Downward-facing dog	38	Hold for 3-5 breaths.	

> continued

Exercise	Page #	Recommended time or reps	Exercise descriptions, recommendations, and variations
Warrior 2 (L)	66	Hold for 3-5 breaths.	
Reverse warrior (L)	68	Hold for 3-5 breaths.	
Extended side angle (L)	70	Hold for 3-5 breaths.	
Half moon (L)	80	Hold for 3-5 breaths.	
Tree pose	76	Hold for 3-5 breaths on each side.	
Transition		Perform a standing forward bend and step back to a kneeling position.	

	Exercise	Page #	Recommended time or reps	Exercise descriptions, recommendations, and variations
Floor fusion exercises (15 min.)	**Two-point tabletop**	92	4-6 reps on each side	Alternate the arm and leg lift and knee to elbow.
	Narrow push-up	88	6-15 reps	Support weight on knees or toes.
	Back extension	94	Hold for 3-5 breaths.	Hands are on the floor.
	Plank with hip drive	86	4-6 reps on each side	
	Upward-facing dog	100	Hold for 3-5 breaths.	If upward-facing dog is uncomfortable, do supported back extension.
	Downward-facing dog	38	Hold for 3-5 breaths.	
	Plank to narrow push-up to upward-facing dog to downward-facing dog	82, 88, 100, 38	1-2 breaths per exercise	Flow dynamically from one exercise to the next in a controlled manner.

> continued

	Exercise	Page #	Recommended time or reps	Exercise descriptions, recommendations, and variations
	Dynamic bow	99	Hold for 3-5 breath each exercise.	Half bow is an option for full bow.
	Wide push-up	89	6-15 reps	Support weight on knees or toes.
	Side twist	110	3-5 reps each side.	Support weight on hand or forearm.
	Full roll-up	103	4-6 reps	
	Abdominal brace position	112	3-5 reps	Hands are behind the head. Curl up and hold for 1-2 breaths, then lower.
	Leg lift tabletop	113	6-10 reps	Lift one leg or both.
	Shoulder bridge position	118	8-10 reps	Lift and lower on a 2-count rhythm.
	Shoulder bridge in external rotation	120	8-10 reps	Lift and lower on a 2-count rhythm.
Calming and restorative exercises (10 min.)	**Reclining knee-hug stretch**	155	Hold for 3-5 breaths.	
	Reclining single-leg hug stretch (R)	156	Hold for 3-5 breaths.	

Exercise	Page #	Recommended time or reps	Exercise descriptions, recommendations, and variations
Reclining hamstring stretch (R)	130	Hold for 3-5 breaths.	
Reclining abductor stretch (R)	141	Hold for 3-5 breaths.	
Reclining adductor stretch (R)	140	Hold for 3-5 breaths.	
Reclining twist (R)	133	Hold for 3-5 breaths.	Keep one leg straight.
Reclining figure-4 (R)	142	Hold for 3-5 breaths.	
Reclining knee-hug stretch	155	Hold for 3-5 breaths.	
Reclining single-leg hug stretch (L)	156	Hold for 3-5 breaths.	
Reclining hamstring stretch (L)	139	Hold for 3-5 breaths.	
Reclining abductor stretch (L)	141	Hold for 3-5 breaths.	

> continued

Exercise	Page #	Recommended time or reps	Exercise descriptions, recommendations, and variations
Reclining adductor stretch (L)	140	Hold for 3-5 breaths.	
Reclining twist (L)	133	Hold for 3-5 breaths.	Keep one leg straight.
Reclining figure-4 (L)	142	Hold for 3-5 breaths.	
Happy baby	158	Hold for 3-5 breaths.	
Calm lake	154	Hold for 5-10 breaths	
Progressive relaxation		Rest for 2-5 min.	

BARRE WORKOUT ☑

This workout is for the dancer in you. The fusion barre workout brings in elements of dance, yoga, and Pilates conditioning. The workout develops endurance, flexibility, balance, and muscle tone. The essence of this workout is to bring grace and fluidity of movement to your workout. Practice the moves with a focus on creating length and extending the limbs as a dancer. You can do the fusion barre workout three or four times per week. Complement this workout with one that is less intense, such as the fusion restoration and relaxation workout. As you develop fitness and skill, increase the tempo of the exercises and choose more challenging variations from the fusion exercises in chapters 4 through 7.

Intention: Even though this workout is challenging, strive for completing the exercises with ease and grace. See yourself as a dancer.

	Exercises	Page #	Recommended time or reps	Exercise descriptions, recommendations, and variations
Warm-up (10 min.)	**Mountain pose with arms reaching**	42	3-4 reps	
	Mountain pose with side bend	43	3-4 reps on each side	
	Dynamic four-point stretch	146	3-4 reps	Move at a controlled pace.

> continued

Barre Workout > *continued*

	Exercises	Page #	Recommended time or reps	Exercise descriptions, recommendations, and variations
	Standing forward bend	41	3-4 reps	Curve the spine and roll down and up in a controlled rhythm.
	Fusion sun salutation flow 1	45	2-3 reps	
	Fusion sun salutation flow 2	46	2-3 reps	
	Fusion sun salutation flow 3	47	2-3 reps	
Transition	**From mountain pose, step out to ballet squat.**			
Standing fusion exercises (20 min.)	**Ballet squat**	58	8-12 reps	

Exercises	Page #	Recommended time or reps	Exercise descriptions, recommendations, and variations
Ballet squat with heel raise	59	8-12 reps	Hold the bottom of the ballet squat and alternate lifting the heels.
Lunge (R)	60	8-12 reps	From the ballet squat, turn to face the side in a lunge stance. From the lunge, lower and stand up on a 2-count rhythm.
Ballet squat	58	8-12 reps	
Ballet squat with heel raise	59	8-12 reps	Hold the bottom of the ballet squat and alternate lifting the heels.
Lunge (L)	60	8-12 reps	From the ballet squat, turn to face the side in a lunge stance. From the lunge, lower and stand up on a 2-count rhythm.
Curtsy squat (R)	57	8-12 reps	

> continued

Exercises	Page #	Recommended time or reps	Exercise descriptions, recommendations, and variations
Curtsy squat (R)	57	8-12 reps	Perform the exercise with rotation.
Side balance (R)	74	Hold for 3-5 breaths.	
Curtsy squat (L)	57	8-12 reps	
Curtsy squat (L)	57	8-12 reps	Perform the exercise with rotation.
Side balance (L)	74	Hold for 3-5 breaths.	

Exercises	Page #	Recommended time or reps	Exercise descriptions, recommendations, and variations
Single-leg balance to lunge (R)	72, 60	8-12 reps	From the single-leg balance, step back to a lunge and return to the knee balance.
Revolving lunge (R)	62	Hold for 3-5 breaths.	
Single-leg balance to lunge (L)	72, 60	8-12 reps	From the single-leg balance, step back to a lunge and return to the knee balance.
Revolving lunge (L)	62	Hold for 3-5 breaths.	

> continued

Barre Workout   *> continued*

	Exercises	Page #	Recommended time or reps	Exercise descriptions, recommendations, and variations
	Curtsy squat to ballet squat (R) 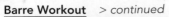	57, 58	8-12 reps	Curtsy squat, step out to a ballet squat, return to curtsy squat, and repeat.
	Curtsy squat to ballet squat (L)	57, 58	8-12 reps	Curtsy squat, step out to ballet squat, return to curtsy squat, and repeat.
	Tree pose	76	Hold for 3-5 breaths on each side.	
Transition	**Perform a standing forward bend and move into a kneeling position.**			
Floor fusion exercises (25 min.)	**Two-point tabletop**	92	4-6 reps of each exercise	Alternate the arm and leg lift and bring knee to elbow. Perform with a leg crossover.
	Breaststroke	96	4-6 reps	

Exercises	Page #	Recommended time or reps	Exercise descriptions, recommendations, and variations
Hip extension	98	4-6 reps	Perform the straight leg or the bend-and-straighten variation.
Dynamic bow	99	Hold for 3-5 breaths.	
Seated forward bend	123	Hold for 3-5 breaths.	Rest in a forward bend before moving on to the next exercises.
V-sit	104	Hold for 3-5 breaths.	Legs are bent, straight, or crossed, and lifted off the floor.
Reverse table	105	Hold for 3-5 breaths.	Use as a transition to a seated position.
Full roll-up	103	4-6 reps	
Bend and stretch	114	4-6 reps	
Single-leg stretch	116	6-10 reps on each side	
Crisscross	117	6-10 reps on each side	
Side bend (R)	109	3-5 reps	

> continued

Exercises	Page #	Recommended time or reps	Exercise descriptions, recommendations, and variations
Side twist (R)	110	3-5 reps	
Side bend (L)	109	3-5 reps	
Side twist (L)	110	3-5 reps	
Shoulder bridge with leg lift	119	8-10 reps	Perform the bent-knee or straight-leg variation.
Shoulder bridge in external rotation	120	8-10 reps	Lift and lower on a 2-count rhythm.
Transition	**Roll up and come to a kneeling position.**		
Calming and restorative exercises (8 min.)	**Kneeling side bend**	150	Hold for 3-5 breaths on each side.	
	Pigeon	137	Hold for 3-5 breaths on each side.	

Exercises	Page #	Recommended time or reps	Exercise descriptions, recommendations, and variations
Seated forward bend	123	Hold for 3-5 breaths.	
Wide-legged forward bend	124	Hold for 3-5 breaths.	
Seated side bend	149	Hold for 3-5 breaths on each side.	
Seated twist	128	Hold for 3-5 breaths on each side.	
Seated butterfly	138	Hold for 3-5 breaths.	
Reclining hamstring stretch (R)	139	Hold for 3-5 breaths.	
Reclining abductor stretch (R)	141	Hold for 3-5 breaths.	
Reclining adductor stretch (R)	140	Hold for 3-5 breaths.	
Reclining knee-hug stretch	155	Hold for 3-5 breaths.	

> continued

Exercises	Page #	Recommended time or reps	Exercise descriptions, recommendations, and variations
Reclining butterfly	157	Hold for 3-5 breaths.	
Reclining hamstring stretch (L)	139	Hold for 3-5 breaths.	
Reclining abductor stretch (L)	141	Hold for 3-5 breaths.	
Reclining adductor stretch (L)	140	Hold for 3-5 breaths.	
Reclining knee-hug stretch	155	Hold for 3-5 breaths.	
Reclining butterfly	157	Hold for 3-5 breaths.	
Resting pose	159	Rest for 2-5 min.	Let go of tension and allow yourself to surrender to the floor. Feel the back of the body sink to the floor. Open the front of the body and allow your breath to move freely through the body.

PILATES CORE WORKOUT

The Pilates core workout will strengthen and define the core and improve alignment. This unique blend of contemporary conditioning, yoga, and Pilates exercises will challenge the core and improve its ability to control movement and generate power. The Pilates core workout is challenging. Give yourself time to progress and take breaks throughout the workout as needed. Do this workout two to four times per week. To make progress in this workout, add more challenging variations from the fusion exercises in chapters 4 through 7.

Intention: Focus on the layers of your core, from the deepest core muscles to the strong outermost muscles. Use the 3D breathing technique to activate the core muscles throughout this workout.

	Exercise	Page #	Recommended time or reps	Exercise descriptions, recommendations, and variations
Warm-up (10 min.)	**Standing 3D breathing**	13	1 min.	Center your mind and body through deep breathing.
	Mountain pose with arms reaching	42	3-4 reps	
	Mountain pose with side bend	43	3-4 reps on each side	

> continued

Pilates Core Workout > continued

Exercise	Page #	Recommended time or reps	Exercise descriptions, recommendations, and variations
Dynamic four-point stretch	146	3-4 reps	Move at a controlled pace.
Standing forward bend	41	3-4 reps	Curve the spine and roll down and up in a slow controlled rhythm.
Fusion sun salutation flow 1	45	2-3 reps	
Fusion sun salutation flow 2	46	2-3 reps	
Low lunge to kneeling hamstring stretch	34	2-3 reps on each side.	Move at a controlled pace.

	Exercise	Page #	Recommended time or reps	Exercise descriptions, recommendations, and variations
Transition	**From the lunge, step up to a standing position.**			
Standing fusion exercises (20 min.)	**Single-leg balance to lunge**	72, 60	8-12 reps on each side	From a single-leg balance, step back into a lunge and then return to a knee balance. Lower and stand up on a 2-count rhythm.
	Side balance	74	Hold for 3-5 breaths on each side.	
	Curtsy squat (R)	57	8-10 reps	Flow from curtsy squat to curtsy squat with rotation. Complete 8-10 reps in both variations.
	Curtsy squat (L)	57	8-10 reps	Flow from curtsy squat to curtsy squat with rotation. Complete 8-10 reps in both variations.

> continued

Exercise	Page #	Recommended time or reps	Exercise descriptions, recommendations, and variations
Crescent lunge to warrior 3 (R)	64, 78	3-5 reps	From crescent lunge, move into warrior 3 and back to crescent lunge on a 2-4 count rhythm.
Warrior 3 (R)	78	Hold for 3-5 breaths.	Hold warrior 3 and move the arms in the swimmer exercise motion.
Crescent lunge to warrior 3 (L)	64, 78	3-5 reps	From crescent lunge, move into warrior 3 and back to crescent lunge on a 2-4 count rhythm.
Warrior 3 (L)	78	Hold for 3-5 breaths.	Hold warrior 3 and move the arms in the swimmer exercise motion.
Ballet squat	58	8-10 reps	Add the heel raise as an option.

	Exercise	Page #	Recommended time or reps	Exercise descriptions, recommendations, and variations
Transition	**Perform a standing forward bend and step back to plank.**			
Floor fusion exercises (25 min.)	**Plank position**	82	Hold for 3-5 breaths.	
	Plank with leg lift	83	6-8 reps on each side	Support the weight on knees or toes. Alternate the leg lifts.
	Narrow push-up	88	4-8 reps	Support the weight on knees or toes.
	Knee-tuck series (R)	84	3-4 reps	
	Knee-tuck series (L)	84	3-4 reps	
	Child's pose	29	Hold for 3-5 breaths.	Rest during this exercise.
	Two-point tabletop	92	Hold each exercise for 3-5 breaths.	Alternate the arm and leg lift and bring opposite knee to elbow.
	Swimmer	95	4-6 reps	
	Breaststroke	96	4-6 reps	
	Side bend (R)	109	3-6 reps	
	Side twist (R)	110	3-6 reps	

> continued

Exercise	Page #	Recommended time or reps	Exercise descriptions, recommendations, and variations
Side bend (L)	109	3-6 reps	
Side twist (L)	110	3-6 reps	
Half rollback	102	6-10 reps	
Half rollback	102	6-10 reps on each side	Perform the oblique variation.
Full roll-up	103	3-6 reps	
Side leg lift (R)	107	4-6 reps	
Side leg circle (R)	108	4-6 reps	
Side leg lift (L)	107	4-6 reps	
Side leg circle (L)	108	4-6 reps	
Abdominal brace position	112	3-4 reps	Hands are behind the head. Curl up, hold for 1-2 breaths, and lower.

	Exercise	Page #	Recommended time or reps	Exercise descriptions, recommendations, and variations
	Bend and stretch	114	6-8 reps on each side	
	Single-leg stretch	116	6-8 reps on each side	
	Crisscross	117	6-8 reps on each side	
	Shoulder bridge with leg lift	119	4-6 reps	Perform the bent-knee or straight-leg option.
Transition	**Come to a kneeling position.**			
Calming and restorative exercises (5 min.)	**Puppy pose**	126	Hold for 3-5 breaths.	
	Supported back extension	144	Hold for 3-5 breaths.	
	Kneeling twist	130	Hold for 3-5 breaths on each side.	

> continued

✓

Exercise	Page #	Recommended time or reps	Exercise descriptions, recommendations, and variations
Thread the needle	132	Hold for 3-5 breaths on each side.	
Kneeling side bend	150	Hold for 3-5 breaths on each side.	
Pigeon	137	Hold for 3-5 breaths on each side.	
Seated forward bend	123	Hold for 3-5 breaths.	
Wide-legged forward bend	124	Hold for 3-5 breaths.	
Crossed-legged seated twist	129	Hold for 3-5 breaths on each side.	
Seated butterfly	138	Hold for 3-5 breaths.	
Seated side bend	149	Hold for 3-5 breaths on each side.	
Happy baby	158	Hold for 5-10 breaths.	

YOGA–PILATES BLEND WORKOUT

This workout uses a perfect blend of yoga and Pilates to build strength, balance, stability, and flexibility. The standing exercises from yoga build strength and stamina, while the Pilates exercises focus on the core. This workout gives you the benefits of both yoga and Pilates in an efficient workout. You can do the fusion yoga–Pilates blend workout three or four times a week and should complement it with the fusion restoration and relaxation workout in chapter 10. To increase the intensity of this workout, add more repetitions of the exercises and hold the static exercises longer. Listen to your body and take breaks when you need to rest.

Intention: Ideally, mobility and stability are perfectly balanced. The exercises in this workout help you find this balance. Observe where you hold tension and lack mobility and assess how this affects your stability. Often when you hold tension or lack mobility, your ability to stabilize is affected. Everyone has body imbalances—take time to notice yours.

	Exercise	Page #	Recommended time or reps	Exercise descriptions, recommendations, and variations
Warm-up (10 min.)	Seated 3D breathing	13	1 min.	Center your mind and body through deep breathing.
	Child's pose	29	Hold for 3-5 breaths.	
	Downward-facing dog	38	Hold for 3-5 breaths.	
	Dynamic four-point stretch	146	3-4 reps	Move at a controlled pace.
	Standing forward bend	41	Hold for 3-5 breaths.	

> continued

Yoga-Pilates Blend Workout > *continued*

	Exercise	Page #	Recommended time or reps	Exercise descriptions, recommendations, and variations
	Fusion sun salutation flow 1	45	2-3 reps	
	Fusion sun salutation flow 2	46	2-3 reps	
	Fusion sun salutation flow 3	47	2-3 reps	
Transition	**From a standing position, step back into a lunge.**			
Standing fusion exercises (20 min.)	**Lunge (R)**	60	8-12 reps	Lower and stand up on a 2-count rhythm.
	Crescent lunge (R)	64	Hold for 3-5 breaths.	

Exercise	Page #	Recommended time or reps	Exercise descriptions, recommendations, and variations
Fusion sun salutation flow 2	46	1-2 breaths per movement	Flow dynamically through these four exercises. Step forward from downward-facing dog to the lunge.
Lunge (L)	60	8-10 reps	Lower and stand up on a 2-count rhythm.
Crescent lunge (L)	64	Hold for 3-5 breaths.	
Fusion sun salutation flow 2	46	1-2 breaths per movement	Flow dynamically through these four exercises. Step forward from downward-facing dog to the warrior 2.
Warrior 2 (R)	66	Hold for 3-5 breaths.	

> continued

Exercise	Page #	Recommended time or reps	Exercise descriptions, recommendations, and variations
Reverse warrior (R)	68	Hold for 3-5 breaths.	
Extended side angle (R)	70	Hold for 3-5 breaths.	
Half moon (R)	80	Hold for 3-5 breaths.	
Fusion sun salutation flow 2	46	1-2 breaths per movement	Flow dynamically through these four exercises. Step forward from downward-facing dog to warrior 2.
Warrior 2 (L)	67	Hold for 3-5 breaths.	

Exercise	Page #	Recommended time or reps	Exercise descriptions, recommendations, and variations
Reverse warrior (L)	68	Hold for 3-5 breaths.	
Extended side angle (L)	70	Hold for 3-5 breaths.	
Half moon (L)	80	Hold for 3-5 breaths.	
Fusion sun salutation flow 2	46	1-2 breaths per movement	Flow dynamically through these four exercises. Step forward from downward-facing dog to warrior 1.
Warrior 1 (R)	65	Hold for 3-5 breaths.	

> continued

Exercise	Page #	Recommended time or reps	Exercise descriptions, recommendations, and variations
Revolving lunge (R)	62	Hold for 3-5 breaths.	Step one foot back to side plank.
Fusion sun salutation flow 2	46	1-2 breaths per movement	Flow dynamically through these four exercises. Step forward from downward-facing dog to warrior 1.
Warrior 1 (L)	65	Hold for 3-5 breaths.	
Revolving lunge (L)	62	Hold for 3-5 breaths.	Step one foot back to side plank.
Squat	50	8-10 reps	

	Exercise	Page #	Recommended time or reps	Exercise descriptions, recommendations, and variations
	Tree pose	76	Hold for 3-5 breaths on each side.	Arms are overhead.
Transition	**Perform a standing forward bend and step back to plank.**			
Floor fusion exercises (25 min.)	**Plank position**	82	Hold for 3-5 breaths.	
	Narrow push-up	88	6-8 reps each side	Support weight on the knees or toes.
	Back extension	94	4-6 reps	
	Side leg lift (R)	107	8-10 reps	
	Side leg circle (R)	108	8-10 reps	
	Side leg lift (L)	107	8-10 reps	
	Side leg circle (L)	108	8-10 reps	
	Dynamic bow	99	4-6 reps on each exercise	Perform the half bow or full bow variation.

> continued

Exercise	Page #	Recommended time or reps	Exercise descriptions, recommendations, and variations
Side twist	110	4-6 reps on each side	
Seated forward bend	123	3-5 breaths	
V-sit	104	3-5 breaths, repeat 2 times.	Legs are bent or straight and lifted off the floor.
Reverse table	105	3-5 breaths, repeat 2 times.	
Full roll-up	103	4-6 reps	
Leg lift tabletop	113	6-10 reps on each side	
Crisscross	117	6-10 reps on each side	
Shoulder bridge with leg lift	119	4-6 reps	Perform the bent-leg or straight-leg option. Lift and lower at a controlled pace.
Transition		**Come to a seated position.**	

	Exercise	Page #	Recommended time or reps	Exercise descriptions, recommendations, and variations
Calming and restorative exercises (8 min.)	**Cross-legged seated forward bend**	125	Hold for 3-5 breaths.	
	Cross-legged seated twist	129	Hold for 3-5 breaths on each side.	
	Seated forward bend	123	Hold for 3-5 breaths.	
	Seated cow face pose	145	Hold for 3-5 breaths on each side.	
	Reclining single leg hug stretch (R)	156	Hold for 3-5 breaths.	
	Reclining hamstring stretch (R)	139	Hold for 3-5 breaths.	
	Reclining figure-4 (R)	142	Hold for 3-5 breaths.	
	Reclining single leg hug stretch (L)	156	Hold for 3-5 breaths.	
	Reclining hamstring stretch (L)	139	Hold for 3-5 breaths.	

> continued

Exercise	Page #	Recommended time or reps	Exercise descriptions, recommendations, and variations
Reclining figure-4 (L)	142	Hold for 3-5 breaths.	
Resting pose	159	Rest for 2-5 min.	Strive for thoughtful meditation. Choose a word that brings you a sense of joy. Focus on your word and the visual images it creates. Your word may be peace, love, gratitude, happy, smile, fulfillment, or whatever you want. Bring this to your life!

Appendix A

Building a Fusion Workout

The fusion workout design template is provided for you to create your own unique fusion workouts. Once you feel confident with the fusion workout exercises, begin to build workouts using the fusion workout five-step system. Simply go back to the chapters for warming up, standing exercises, floor exercises, and calming and restorative exercises and choose what you will do for your workout.

Fill in your exercise selections, duration, and repetitions in the blank fusion workout template. The number of exercises you select is based on your skill level, fitness, time available, and exercise preferences. The length of time you hold an exercise or the number of repetitions you perform is based on your workout intention, whether it is a challenging workout or a restorative workout, and the objective you want to accomplish. In other words, if you want to challenge yourself, you need to complete enough repetitions or hold the exercise long enough to feel muscle fatigue. If your objective is to restore, choose fewer exercises from the standing and floor strength, balance, and flexibility and more exercises from the calming and restorative section.

As a general guideline, select four or five exercises for warming up or do the fusion sun salutation, five to eight exercises for standing and floor strength, balance, and flexibility and finish with four or five exercises from calming and restorative. Vary the tempo, number of repetitions, and length of holds to give you a suitable workout.

Be creative and try different exercise combinations, or use one of the fusion workouts provided for ideas and add or change some of the exercises to enhance variety. For example, start with alternating fitness lunges for 10 repetitions, then hold a yoga crescent lunge for five deep breaths on your right leg, move into a yoga warrior 3 pose for five deep breaths, and finish with fitness squats for 10 repetitions. Repeat the sequence of exercises on the left side, beginning with the fitness lunges.

Your fusion workout options are endless. Have fun experimenting with your workouts, but always remember to be safe. Move in a pain-free range of motion and select exercises that are appropriate for you. The number of repetitions you choose should be challenging, but not exhausting. When holding an exercise, remember to use the 3D breathing technique to provide the body with much-needed energy and focus.

FUSION FIVE-STEP SYSTEM WORKOUT TEMPLATE

Intention: _____

	Exercise	Page #	Recommended time or reps.	Exercise recommendations and variations
Warm-up (5 min.)				

Transition

	Exercise	Page #	Recommended time or reps.	Exercise recommendations and variations
Standing fusion exercises (10 min.)				

Transition

	Exercise	Page #	Recommended time or reps.	Exercise recommendations and variations
Floor fusion exercises (10 min.)				

Transition

	Exercise	Page #	Recommended time or reps.	Exercise recommendations and variations
Calming and restorative exercises (5 min.)				

From H. Vanderburg, 2017, *Fusion Workouts*. (Champaign, IL: Human Kinetics).

Appendix B

Sample Weekly Fusion Workout Plans

The sample fusion workout plans are suggested weekly workouts that progress over six weeks. The workouts are intentionally performed daily to create an exercise habit and are balanced between harder and easier workout days. Take the first week of each progression to get accustomed to the exercises and workouts. In the second week, challenge yourself to improve your technique, mindfulness or to perform more advanced versions of the fusion exercises. Once you complete the full six-week progression, you can circle back to weeks 3 and 4 or move on to the next level.

Beginner

At the beginner level, start each workout with breath awareness and 3D breathing exercises. As well, practice simple mediation two or three times per week during weeks 1 and 2; three or four times per week during weeks 3 and 4; and four or five times per week during weeks 5 and 6. This can be done before or after your workout or at a separate time.

BEGINNER   WEEKS 1 AND 2

Monday	Pg. 164	Begin level workout
Tuesday	Pg. 190	20-minute workout
Wednesday	Pg. 245	Restoration and relaxation workout
Thursday	Pg. 164	Begin level workout
Friday	Pg. 190	20-minute workout
Saturday	Pg. 245	Restoration and relaxation workout
Sunday	Pg. 210	Core conditioning workout

BEGINNER   WEEKS 3 AND 4

Monday	Pg. 164	Begin level workout
Tuesday	Pg. 228	Upper-body conditioning workout
Wednesday	Pg. 236	Lower-body conditioning workout
Thursday	Pg. 245	Restoration and relaxation workout
Friday	Pg. 210	Core conditioning workout
Saturday	Pg. 190	20-minute workout
Sunday	Pg. 245	Restoration and relaxation workout

BEGINNER   WEEKS 5 AND 6

Monday	Pg. 169	Evolve level workout
Tuesday	Pg. 245	Restoration and relaxation workout
Wednesday	Pg. 210	Core conditioning workout
Thursday	Pg. 228	Upper-body conditioning workout
Friday	Pg. 261	Barre workout
Saturday	Pg. 245	Restoration and relaxation workout
Sunday	Pg. 190	20-minute workout

Intermediate

At the intermediate level, start each workout with breath awareness and 3D breathing exercises. Practice simple mediation two or three times per week during weeks 1 and 2; three or four times per week during weeks 3 and 4; and four or five times per week during weeks 5 and 6.

INTERMEDIATE   WEEKS 1 AND 2

Monday	Pg. 169	Evolve level workout
Tuesday	Pg. 210	Core conditioning workout
Wednesday	Pg. 195	40-minute workout
Thursday	Pg. 245	Restoration and relaxation workout
Friday	Pg. 279	Yoga-Pilates blend workout
Saturday	Pg. 169	Evolve level workout
Sunday	Pg. 245	Restoration and relaxation workout

INTERMEDIATE   WEEKS 3 AND 4

Monday	Pg. 195	40-minute workout
Tuesday	Pg. 169	Evolve level workout
Wednesday	Pg. 261	Barre workout
Thursday	Pg. 245	Restoration and relaxation workout
Friday	Pg. 228	Upper-body conditioning workout
Saturday	Pg. 236	Lower-body conditioning workout
Sunday	Pg. 245	Restoration and relaxation workout

INTERMEDIATE   WEEKS 5 AND 6

Monday	Pg. 220	Full-body conditioning workout
Tuesday	Pg. 271	Pilates core workout
Wednesday	Pg. 195	40-minute workout
Thursday	Pg. 245	Restoration and relaxation workout
Friday	Pg. 279	Yoga-Pilates blend workout
Saturday	Pg. 169	Evolve level workout
Sunday	Pg. 245	Restoration and relaxation workout

Advanced

At the advanced level, start each workout with breath awareness and 3D breathing exercises. Practice simple mediation two or three times per week during weeks 1 and 2; three or four times per week during weeks 3 and 4; and four or five times per week during weeks 5 and 6.

ADVANCED   WEEKS 1 AND 2

Monday	Pg. 177	Challenge level workout
Tuesday	Pg. 271	Pilates core workout
Wednesday	Pg. 200	60-minute workout
Thursday	Pg. 261	Barre workout
Friday	Pg. 245	Restoration and relaxation workout
Saturday	Pg. 220	Full-body conditioning workout
Sunday	Pg. 210	Core conditioning workout

ADVANCED   WEEKS 3 AND 4

Monday	Pg. 252	Athlete workout
Tuesday	Pg. 279	Yoga-Pilates blend workout
Wednesday	Pg. 200	60-minute workout
Thursday	Pg. 245	Restoration and relaxation workout
Friday	Pg. 220	Full-body conditioning workout
Saturday	Pg. 177	Challenge level workout
Sunday	Pg. 271	Pilates core workout

ADVANCED   WEEKS 5 AND 6

Monday	Pg. 220	Full-body conditioning workout
Tuesday	Pg. 261	Barre workout
Wednesday	Pg. 177	Challenge level workout
Thursday	Pg. 200	60-minute workout
Friday	Pg. 271	Pilates core workout
Saturday	Pg. 252	Athlete workout
Sunday	Pg. 245	Restoration and relaxation workout